# Abbreviations and glossary

**ACE:** angiotensin-converting enzyme

**ADH:** antidiuretic hormone

**AKI:** acute kidney injury; a sudden reduction in glomerular filtration rate, resulting in the accumulation of fluid and nitrogenous waste products

**Albuminuria/microalbuminuria:** the presence of albumin in the urine; microalbuminuria is a slight increase in urinary albumin levels that provides an early marker for kidney disease

**AML:** angiomyolipoma

**ANCA:** antineutrophil cytoplasm antibody

**APKD:** autosomal-dominant polycystic kidney disease

**ARB:** angiotensin-receptor blocker

**ASA:** acetylsalicylic acid; aspirin

**ATN:** acute tubular necrosis

**Bacteriuria:** the presence of bacteria in the urine

**BPH:** benign prostatic hyperplasia

**BUN:** blood urea nitrogen (also known as serum urea)

**C-ANCA:** cytoplasmic antineutrophil cytoplasm antibody

**CKD:** chronic kidney disease; the presence of kidney damage for at least 3 months, with either structural or functional abnormalities of the kidney with or without decreased glomerular filtration rate

**CT:** computerized tomography

**ECG:** electrocardiogram

**ESA:** erythropoiesis-stimulating agent

**ESKD:** end-stage kidney disease

**ESR:** erythrocyte sedimentation rate

**ESWL:** extracorporeal shock-wave lithotripsy

**GBM:** glomerular basement membrane

**GFR:** glomerular filtration rate; the volume of fluid filtered from the plasma through glomerular capillary walls in the kidney into the Bowman's capsule per unit time

**Glomerulonephritis:** inflammation of the glomeruli (small filtering units) in the kidney

**GPA:** granulomatosis with polyangiitis

**Hematuria:** the presence of erythrocytes (red blood cells) in the urine

**HIV:** human immunodeficiency virus

**HUS:** hemolytic uremic syndrome

**Ig:** immunoglobulin

**Interstitial nephritis:** inflammation of the interstitium of the kidney surrounding the tubules

**LDL:** low-density lipoprotein

**MCGN:** mesangiocapillary glomerulonephritis

**MDRD:** modification of diet in renal disease

**NSAIDs:** non-steroidal anti-inflammatory drugs

**Oliguria/anuria:** the low output/no output of urine

**P-ANCA:** perinuclear antineutrophil cytoplasm antibody

**Proteinuria:** the presence of excess serum proteins in the urine

**PTH:** parathyroid hormone

**SIADH:** syndrome of inappropriate secretion of ADH

**SLE:** systemic lupus erythematosus; a long-term autoimmune disorder that affects the joints, skin, nervous system and kidneys

**TTP:** thrombotic thrombocytopenic purpura

**UTI:** urinary tract infection

**Uremia:** an excess of urea and other nitrogenous waste in the blood

# Introduction

Kidney disease is common and its prevalence is increasing worldwide. Up to 8% of the population of developed countries has some degree of renal impairment; in the USA, over 19 million adults have some form of chronic kidney disease (CKD) and 1 in 1000 is receiving treatment for end-stage kidney disease (ESKD). It is estimated that the direct medical costs of ESKD exceed US$30 billion per year in the USA; the total cost of dialysis is over US$77 000/patient/year in the UK.

CKD is often a progressive condition, but the rate of decline can be slowed and complications can be substantially reduced by timely treatment. This is especially important for the increasing number of patients with diabetes and hypertension in whom treatment can greatly reduce morbidity. Specific treatment is now available for many patients with glomerulonephritis, a common cause of CKD.

Since most patients will not be seen by nephrologists, CKD needs to be effectively managed by community and family doctors. While this has improved in the last few years, many patients still do not receive appropriate treatments early in CKD.

Acute kidney injury (AKI) is significantly less common, but still affects 5% of hospitalized patients. Although it is an important cause of morbidity and mortality, and can lead to CKD, it can often be treated successfully; however, it is increasingly clear that many patients with AKI are not well managed. Depressingly, a recent UK national audit indicated that only 50% of patients with AKI received 'good' care (under non-nephrologists); there is therefore much room for improvement in the proper management of AKI, much of which is based on sound clinical medicine, including management of volume status, drug chart review, and repeated and appropriate investigations.

It is therefore important for all physicians, both in hospitals and the community, to have an awareness of renal disease, its management and its complications. We hope this second edition of *Fast Facts: Renal Disorders* will help to achieve this.

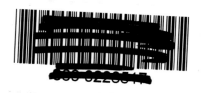

# Fast Facts:
# Renal Disorders

**DATE DUE**

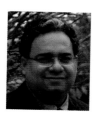

### Ajay Singh MBBS FRCP MBA
Director, Global Programs
Associate Professor of Medicine
Harvard Medical School
Physician, Renal Division
Brigham and Women's Hospital, Boston, MA, USA

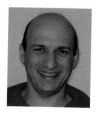

### Jeremy Levy MA PhD FHEA FRCP
Consultant Nephrologist
Imperial College Healthcare NHS Trust
London, UK

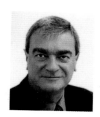

### Charles Pusey DSc FRCP FRCPath FMedSci
Professor of Medicine
Head of Renal Section, Department of Medicine
Imperial College London
London, UK

**Declaration of Independence**
This book is as balanced and as practical as we can make it.
Ideas for improvement are always welcome: feedback@fastfacts.com

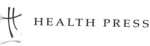
HEALTH PRESS

Fast Facts: Renal Disorders
First published February 2006
Second edition June 2013

Health Press Limited, Elizabeth House, Queen Street, Abingdon,
Oxford OX14 3LN, UK
Tel: +44 (0)1235 523233
Fax: +44 (0)1235 523238

Book orders can be placed by telephone or via the website.
For regional distributors or to order via the website, please go to:
www.fastfacts.com
For telephone orders, please call +44 (0)1752 202301 (UK, Europe and Asia–
Pacific), 1 800 247 6553 (USA, toll free) or +1 419 281 1802 (Americas).

Fast Facts is a trademark of Health Press Limited.

A CIP record for this title is available from the British Library.

ISBN 978-1-908541-18-5

Singh A (Ajay)
Fast Facts: Renal Disorders/
Ajay Singh, Jeremy Levy, Charles Pusey

Medical illustrations by Dee McLean, London, UK.
Typesetting and page layout by Zed, Oxford, UK.
Printed by Latimer Trend & Company Limited, Plymouth, UK.

Text printed with vegetable inks on biodegradable and recyclable
paper manufactured using elemental chlorine free (ECF) wood
pulp from well-managed forests.

FSC
www.fsc.org
MIX
Paper from
responsible sources
FSC® C013436

The clinical symptoms of renal disease often do not become apparent until kidney failure is advanced. Screening for renal disease is, therefore, particularly important, because it may enable abnormalities to be detected in time for effective treatment to be started. Bedside urine analysis is an essential part of any clinical examination. Urine testing may also be part of a routine medical examination for insurance or employment purposes, or when a person registers with a new primary care physician.

Urinary abnormalities will be found in most patients with renal disease, particularly positive dipstick tests for blood or protein, or the presence of cells, casts, crystals or organisms on urine microscopy. Clinically, severe hematuria may be reported if the patient has red or dark urine, which, if it occurs at the end of the urinary stream, suggests bleeding from the lower urinary tract. Heavy proteinuria can produce unusually frothy urine, but this is not often reported spontaneously.

## Proteinuria

Proteinuria may originate from anywhere within the urinary tract. High levels of protein in the urine (> 3 g/day) generally reflect the presence of albuminuria and point to a glomerular process (glomerular albuminuria). Proteinuria due to tubular damage is usually only low level (< 1 g/day) and involves proteins of a lower molecular weight, such as β2-microglobulin. Overflow proteinuria may result from the filtration of abnormal amounts of low-molecular-weight proteins through the glomeruli, such as monoclonal light chains in myeloma.

One of the most common causes of low-level proteinuria is inflammation in the lower urinary tract, which is usually caused by urinary tract infection (UTI) (Table 1.1). Women are at increased risk of UTI because of renal tract dilatation leading to urinary stasis, and this should be treated promptly according to bacterial sensitivity.

Urinary protein excretion increases during pregnancy, but never to more than 300 mg/day, so overt proteinuria is not physiological.

TABLE 1.1
**Causes of proteinuria**

**Glomerular proteinuria (most common cause)**
- Primary glomerulonephritis of all histological types
- Secondary glomerular disease due to diabetes, systemic lupus erythematosus or amyloidosis

**Tubular proteinuria**
- Tubulointerstitial nephritis, often related to drugs, but with many other causes
- Toxins, such as heavy metals and tetracycline, damaging the tubule

**Overflow proteinuria**
- Multiple myeloma and monoclonal immunoglobulin deposition disease
- Myoglobinuria
- Hemoglobinuria

**Tissue proteinuria**
- Acute inflammation of the urinary tract
- Urinary tract tumors

**Dipstick testing** of the urine is designed to detect albumin and is insensitive to other proteins; it will not, therefore, generally detect light chains in myeloma. Dipsticks may detect albumin concentrations as low as 20–30 mg/dL, and are often calibrated on a scale of 0–3+, which provides a semiquantitative estimate of protein concentration. Highly concentrated urine may produce false-positive results, while dilute urine may produce false-negative results.

**Timed and spot urine samples.** Proteinuria may be formally quantified using timed urine samples, usually a 24-hour specimen. The upper end of the normal range is 150 mg/24 hours. As collecting 24-hour urine samples is difficult and unreliable, measurement of the albumin:creatinine or protein:creatinine ratio from a spot urine sample is increasingly being used, because it correlates well with 24-hour albumin or protein excretion. In conventional units an albumin:creatinine ratio of 1 equates to 1 g/24 hours of albumin excretion, and in SI units a ratio of 120 mg/mmol equates to 1 g/24 hours albuminuria. Albuminuria of more than 1 g/24 hours, in the absence of an obvious cause, should prompt further investigation, which might include kidney biopsy. Albuminuria of more than 3.5 g/24 hours is commonly associated with nephrotic syndrome (see Chapter 6).

## Hematuria

Whereas significant albuminuria often indicates intrinsic renal parenchymal disease, hematuria may be caused by lesions throughout the urinary tract, particularly infection or malignancy (Table 1.2).

Several clinical algorithms have been proposed for the investigation of hematuria (Figure 1.1). In general, once UTI has been excluded, then hematuria *without* significant proteinuria should prompt a search for malignancy in older patients, while hematuria with proteinuria requires a search for a glomerular cause.

**Dipstick testing** of the urine provides a semiquantitative estimate of the degree of hematuria, but hemoglobin (in hemolysis) and myoglobin (in rhabdomyolysis) may also produce positive tests.

**Urine microscopy** should always be performed to detect red blood cells. Misshapen or dysmorphic red cells, detected by an experienced observer using phase-contrast microscopy, suggest glomerular hematuria. The presence of red-cell or granular casts in the urine is a more reliable way of identifying a renal source of the hematuria, as opposed to a ureteric or bladder source. Red-cell casts, in particular, generally indicate active glomerulonephritis. In most cases, significant albuminuria in addition to hematuria is seen in glomerular disease.

## Kidney function tests

Kidney function is assessed most simply by measuring the serum concentrations of metabolites excreted by the kidney, most commonly urea and creatinine. The serum urea concentration is influenced more by dietary intake of protein, the state of hydration, liver function and various drugs. Serum creatinine is, therefore, a more reliable measure, but is related directly to muscle mass; thus, a small elderly woman may have a

TABLE 1.2

**Causes of hematuria**

**Glomerular disease**
- Most types of primary glomerulonephritis (rare in membranous and minimal change disease)
- Secondary glomerulonephritis due to systemic vasculitis, systemic lupus erythematosus, Goodpasture's syndrome, Henoch–Schönlein purpura or postinfectious nephritis
- Hereditary nephritis, such as Alport's syndrome and thin basement membrane disease

**Disease of the interstitium or tubule**
- Acute interstitial nephritis, particularly due to drugs
- Hereditary disease, such as polycystic kidney disease and medullary sponge kidney
- Vascular disorders, such as malignant hypertension and renal artery embolism (including cholesterol emboli)
- Papillary necrosis due to diabetes, sickle-cell disease and analgesic abuse

**Disease of the renal pelvis, ureter and bladder**
- Transitional cell carcinoma
- Bladder carcinoma
- Calculi
- Infection (e.g. tuberculosis, schistosomiasis)
- Acute inflammation (e.g. urinary tract infection)
- Toxins (e.g. cyclophosphamide)
- Trauma

**Coagulation disturbances**
- Abnormalities of the coagulation system or platelets (many inherited and acquired disorders)

normal serum creatinine with a markedly reduced glomerular filtration rate (GFR). Changes in serum creatinine (especially a rise) can be a useful guide to deteriorating kidney function; absolute values do not correlate well with GFR.

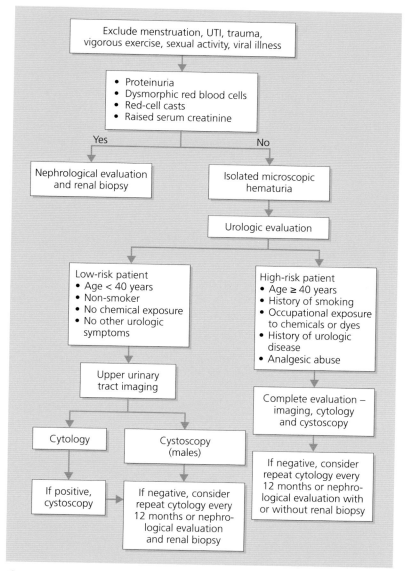

**Figure 1.1** An algorithm for the investigation of hematuria.

**Serum creatinine in pregnancy.** During a normal pregnancy in a woman with normal kidneys, renal plasma flow and GFR both increase (by ≥ 50%), leading to a reduction in the mean serum creatinine during the

11

first and second trimesters from 73 µmol/L (0.8 mg/dL) to 51 µmol/L (0.5 mg/dL). No fall in serum creatinine during pregnancy can indicate significant renal functional impairment.

Women with only mild renal impairment from any cause will usually have a successful pregnancy outcome, and will seldom incur any additional kidney damage as a result of the pregnancy. Some women, however, will have complications during the pregnancy itself, especially hypertension (see pages 64–6). Women with more severe renal impairment are more likely to suffer hypertension, pre-eclampsia or premature labor, and to have a small baby, miscarriage or irreversible decline in renal function in the long term (Table 1.3).

**Measurement of glomerular filtration rate.** Creatinine clearance, which assesses creatinine excretion over 24 hours in relation to the serum creatinine level, is often used as a measure of GFR. However, it can overestimate GFR, since up to 25% of urinary creatinine may come from tubular secretion, and 24-hour urine collections are unreliable. It is also important to realize that a significant rise in serum creatinine does not occur until the GFR is reduced to about 50% of normal.

A number of formulas have been described to estimate GFR based on the serum creatinine and characteristics of the patient (e.g. age, weight, sex, race). The three best-known formulas are the Cockcroft–Gault equation, the Modification of Diet in Renal Disease study (MDRD)

TABLE 1.3

**Pregnancy outcomes for women with pre-existing renal disease**

| Creatinine level | Problems during pregnancy | Successful obstetric outcome | Long-term problems |
|---|---|---|---|
| < 125 µmol/L (1.4 mg/dL) | 26% | 96% | < 3% |
| 125–250 µmol/L (1.4–2.8 mg/dL) | 47% | 89% | 25% |
| > 250 µmol/L (2.8 mg/dL) | 88% | 46% | 53% |

equation and the chronic kidney disease (CKD)-Epi formula (Table 1.4). The MDRD and CKD-Epi formulas are more precise measures of kidney function and have been widely adopted by hospital-based and commercial

TABLE 1.4

**Formulas for calculating creatinine clearance or glomerular filtration rate**

Cockcroft–Gault formula (SI units)

$(140 - \text{age}) \times$ weight (kg)/SCr (μmol/L) $\times$ 1.23 if male or $\times$ 1.04 if female

Cockcroft–Gault (conventional units)

$[(140 - \text{age}) \times$ weight (kg)/SCr (mg/dL) $\times$ 72] if male $\times$ 0.85 if female

MDRD formula (SI units)

$170 \times (\text{SCr [μmol/L]} \times 0.0114)^{-0.999} \times \text{age}^{-0.176} \times (\text{BUN} \times 2.8)^{-0.17} \times \text{albumin}^{0.318} \times 0.762$ if female $\times$ 1.18 if black

MDRD formula (conventional units)

$170 \times \text{SCr (mg/dL)}^{-0.999} \times \text{age}^{-0.176} \times \text{BUN}^{-0.17} \times \text{albumin}^{0.318} \times 0.762$ if female $\times$ 1.18 if black

MDRD formula – brief version (SI units)

$186 \times (\text{SCr [mmol/L]} \times 0.0114)^{-1.154} \times \text{age}^{-0.203} \times 0.742$ if female $\times$ 1.21 if black

MDRD formula – brief version (conventional units)

$186 \times \text{SCr (mg/dL)}^{-1.154} \times \text{age}^{-0.203} \times 0.742$ if female $\times$ 1.21 if black

CKD-EPI equation

$\text{eGFR} = 141 \times \min(\text{SCr[mg/dL]}/k, 1)^{a} \times \max(\text{SCr}/k, 1)^{-1.209} \times 0.993^{\text{Age}} \times [1.018 \text{ if female}] \times [1.159 \text{ if black}]$

where k is 0.7 for females and 0.9 for males, a is –0.329 for females and –0.411 for males, min indicates the minimum of SCr/k or 1, and max indicates the maximum of SCr/k or 1.

BUN, blood urea nitrogen (serum urea); CKD, chronic kidney disease; GFR, glomerular filtration rate; MDRD, modification of diet in renal disease; SCr, serum creatinine.

laboratories. Newer methods, which may find their way into clinical practice, include iohexol clearance and serum cystatin concentration.

## Other blood tests

The diagnosis of many renal diseases is assisted by specific blood tests, particularly in glomerular disease. These tests include measurement of blood glucose for diabetes mellitus, and serum electrophoresis for myeloma and other B-cell dyscrasias. It should be noted that in pregnancy, glycosuria is common and does not usually indicate diabetes or even impaired glucose tolerance.

A range of immunologic tests (e.g. anti-DNA antibodies and complement levels in systemic lupus erythematosus [SLE]) is helpful in the diagnosis of glomerulonephritis.

## Kidney imaging

The investigation of renal disease should always include some form of kidney imaging, which can provide both anatomic and functional information (Table 1.5). In general, it is appropriate to start with cheaper, non-invasive methods of imaging, such as ultrasonography, and use more invasive and expensive methods selectively.

## Kidney biopsy

Percutaneous kidney biopsy can provide a definitive histological diagnosis of glomerular or interstitial disease. It is particularly helpful in patients with severe proteinuria, hematuria that is not due to disease of the lower urinary tract, and acute kidney failure thought to be caused by intrinsic renal disease (rather than prerenal disease, obstruction or acute tubular necrosis [ATN]). The main diseases diagnosed by kidney biopsy include glomerulonephritis, glomerular disorders such as amyloid and diabetes, and interstitial nephritis. Opinions differ as to when a kidney biopsy is indicated, but the potential benefit in terms of treatment usually outweighs the risk involved (significant bleeding in about 1 in 1000 cases). If both kidneys are small, as in chronic glomerulonephritis, then the risk generally outweighs the benefit. In the presence of microscopic hematuria alone, or albuminuria of less than 1 g/24 hours, kidney biopsy is often not indicated since it is unlikely that a specific treatment would be required. However,

higher levels of albuminuria or the combination of albuminuria and

TABLE 1.5

**Kidney imaging techniques**

| Indication | Major advantages |
|---|---|
| **Ultrasonography** | |
| • Estimates kidney size (differentiates acute from chronic kidney disease) | • Cheap |
| | • Easy to perform |
| • Detects structural abnormalities (e.g. cysts, reflux) | • Portable |
| • Excludes obstruction | |
| • Guides biopsy or nephrostomy | |
| **Doppler ultrasonography** | |
| • Screens for renal artery stenosis or thrombosis | • Cheap |
| | • Reliable if good Doppler signals obtained |
| **Computerized tomography** | |
| • Provides detailed anatomic information about the kidneys | • Good anatomic detail |
| • Examines ureters and bladder | |
| **Magnetic resonance imaging** | |
| • Provides anatomic information about the kidneys | • Nephrotoxic contrast not used |
| • Examines ureters and bladder | |
| • Defines renovascular lesions | |
| **Radionucleotide imaging** | |
| • Provides functional information about each kidney | • Nephrotoxic contrast not used |
| • Screens for renovascular disease (with captopril) or obstruction (with furosemide) | |
| • Obtains quantitative functional data | |
| **Renal angiography** | |
| • Gold standard for detection of renovascular disorders including renal artery stenosis and aneurysms | • Excellent definition of vascular anatomy and opportunity for intervention |
| • Provides intervention for angioplasty, stenting or embolization | |

hematuria (particularly with casts) are indications for biopsy, because a number of causes of glomerulonephritis (see Chapter 6) and interstitial nephritis are now amenable to therapy.

## Key points – proteinuria, hematuria and renal investigations

- Proteinuria and hematuria should always be investigated.
- Proteinuria should be quantified by means of an albumin:creatinine ratio or 24-hour collections, since the result will guide management.
- Hematuria may have a medical or surgical cause, and this should be assessed before starting investigations.
- Serum creatinine alone is an unreliable guide to kidney function; an assessment of glomerular filtration rate is more useful.
- No fall in serum creatinine during pregnancy can indicate significant renal functional impairment.

### Key references

Baylis C. Impact of pregnancy on underlying renal disease. *Adv Ren Replace Ther* 2003;10:31–9.

Jayne D. Hematuria and proteinuria. In: *Primer on Kidney Disease*, 5th edn, Greenberg A (ed). Philadelphia: Saunders Elsevier, 2009:33–42.

Johnson CA, Levey AS, Coresh J et al. Clinical practice guidelines for chronic kidney disease in adults: Part II. Glomerular filtration rate, proteinuria, and other markers. *Am Fam Physician* 2004;70:1091–7.

Margulis V, Sagalowsky AI. Assessment of hematuria. *Med Clin North Am* 2011;95:153–9.

Sanders CL, Lucas MJ. Renal disease in pregnancy. *Obstet Gynecol Clin North Am* 2001;28:593–600.

# 2 Electrolyte disturbances and acid–base disorders

Plasma electrolyte and acid–base disturbances are common clinical problems. Perturbations may result in morbidity and mortality, particularly in the elderly and young children, and in those with other comorbid states, such as sepsis, coronary heart disease and heart failure.

## Sodium and water disorders

Regulation of the plasma sodium concentration by the body relies on:
- the balance between intake and excretion of both sodium and water
- the function of sensors of osmolality and extracellular fluid volume (e.g. hypothalamic osmoreceptors, carotid baroreceptors)
- effector mechanisms such as antidiuretic hormone (ADH) and aldosterone.

**Hyponatremia.** Mild hyponatremia (plasma sodium 130–135 mmol/L) is common and affects approximately 15–20% of hospitalized patients. More severe hyponatremia (plasma sodium < 130 mmol/L) is rarer and occurs in less than 1–4% of patients (Table 2.1).

*Clinical features.* Hyponatremia in conjunction with hypo-osmolality (as is common) causes clinical problems, especially when the plasma sodium concentration falls below 120 mmol/L, and patients usually complain of nausea and malaise. When the plasma sodium reaches 115 mmol/L, patients may complain of headache and become delirious. Seizures and coma are common when the plasma sodium falls below 110 mmol/L. These neurological complications reflect water shifting osmotically into the brain. Premenopausal women and children seem to be particularly susceptible to symptomatic hyponatremia for reasons that are unclear.

*Diagnosis* of hypo-osmolar hyponatremia requires careful assessment of extracellular volume and measurement of urinary sodium to determine whether total body sodium is low, normal or high. Adrenal failure, kidney failure and hypothyroidism must always be excluded.

The history and physical examination should focus on identifying any underlying cause of the hyponatremia, such as a malignancy causing a

17

TABLE 2.1

**Causes of hyponatremia and hypo-osmolality**

**Hypovolemic hyponatremia (reduction in total body sodium)**
- Renal losses – diuretics, hypoaldosteronism, salt-wasting nephropathy
- Gastrointestinal – vomiting, diarrhea, enteral tube drainage
- Skin – excessive sweating, burns

**Euvolemic hyponatremia (normal total body sodium)**
- Syndrome of inappropriate antidiuretic hormone secretion
- Cortisol deficiency
- Kidney failure
- Hypothyroidism
- Pregnancy
- Pyschosis
- Primary polydipsia

**Hypervolemic hyponatremia (increased total body sodium)**
- Heart failure
- Nephrotic syndrome
- Cirrhosis

syndrome of inappropriate secretion of ADH (SIADH). Investigations should confirm hypo-osmolality, and demonstrate either appropriate or inappropriate secretion of ADH by comparing urine osmolality with plasma osmolality. Urine osmolality below 100 mOsmol/kg (i.e. very dilute urine) indicates that ADH secretion is completely and appropriately suppressed. Urine osmolality above 100 mOsmol/kg, and particularly in the range of 200–600 mOsmol/kg, usually indicates inappropriate secretion of ADH. A diagnosis of SIADH can be easily made based on specific diagnostic criteria (Tables 2.2 and 2.3).

*Treatment.* Particular care must be taken when correcting hyponatremia in premenopausal women, children and those with very low plasma sodium levels (< 120 mmol/L). Severe symptomatic hyponatremia may require treatment with hypertonic (3%) sodium chloride. The sodium concentration should be monitored frequently. The optimal correction rate should be

TABLE 2.2

**Common disorders associated with the syndrome of inappropriate antidiuretic hormone secretion**

| Pulmonary | Neurological |
|---|---|
| • Abscess | • Neoplasm |
| • Tuberculosis | • Head trauma |
| • Pneumonia | • Encephalitis |
| • Aspergillosis | • Meningitis |
| • Positive-pressure ventilation | • Brain abscess |
| • Asthma | • Guillain–Barré syndrome |

Neoplastic

| • Lung | • Stomach |
|---|---|
| • Pancreas | • Prostate |
| • Lymphoma | • Bladder |

TABLE 2.3

**Diagnostic criteria for syndrome of inappropriate antidiuretic hormone secretion**

• Hyponatremia and hypo-osmolality
• Normal extracellular volume
• Urine osmolality > 100 mOsmol/kg
• Urine sodium > 20 mmol/L
• Normal kidney, adrenal, hepatic and thyroid function

0.5–1 mmol/L/hour, with a total correction of plasma sodium of 10–12 mmol over the first 24 hours. A more aggressive correction rate of 2.0 mmol/L/hour may be considered in patients with seizures or severe neurological symptoms attributable to hyponatremia. However, an overly rapid correction rate carries the risk of precipitating central pontine myelinolysis.

Vasopressin receptor antagonists are a new class of agents developed for selective use in the treatment of hyponatremia, especially in patients with SIADH, congestive heart failure or liver cirrhosis. These 'vaptan' drugs (conivaptan and tolvaptan) have been specifically developed to inhibit the action of vasopressin on its receptors (V1A, V1B and V2). However, their precise clinical role has yet to be elucidated.

**Hypernatremia** (plasma sodium concentration ≥ 145 mmol/L) is common among hospitalized patients, particularly the elderly. Hypernatremia is also often seen in individuals who have lost their perception of thirst (e.g. as a result of a neurological disability) or who have been denied free access to water (Table 2.4). Hypernatremia always reflects a state of hyperosmolality. Since sodium is usually confined to the extracellular space, an actual or relative increase in sodium (compared with water) results in the movement of water out of cells driven by osmosis. Cellular dehydration follows, and shrinkage of brain cells causes most of the clinical manifestations.

*Clinical features.* Mild hypernatremia (plasma sodium 150–155 mmol/L) is usually associated with nausea, vomiting, irritability and a depressed sensorium. More severe hypernatremia (plasma sodium > 160 mmol/L) may result in seizures, focal neurological defects, stupor and coma. In

TABLE 2.4

**Causes of hypernatremia and hyperosmolality**

**Hypovolemic hypernatremia (reduction in total body sodium)**
- Skin – burns, excessive sweating
- Gastrointestinal – diarrhea, vomiting

**Euvolemic hypernatremia (normal total body sodium)**
- Skin – burns, excessive sweating
- Respiratory – tachypnea
- Renal losses
- Central diabetes insipidus
- Nephrogenic diabetes insipidus

**Hypervolemic hypernatremia (increased total body sodium)**
- Hypertonic parenteral nutrition
- Hypertonic saline or sodium bicarbonate administration

children, muscle spasticity, fever and labored respiration may be prominent.

The speed with which hypernatremia develops also appears to modulate the severity of the clinical features. Severe, acute hypernatremia may result in irreversible vascular damage, particularly in children. Acute hypernatremia is associated with a mortality of 40%, whereas chronic hypernatremia is associated with a mortality of 10%.

*Diagnosis.* The differential diagnosis of hypernatremia requires an initial assessment of extracellular volume (Figure 2.1). The history and physical examination should focus on identifying any underlying cause.

*Treatment.* Hypovolemic hypernatremic patients can be managed by administration of isotonic saline. Patients with hypervolemic

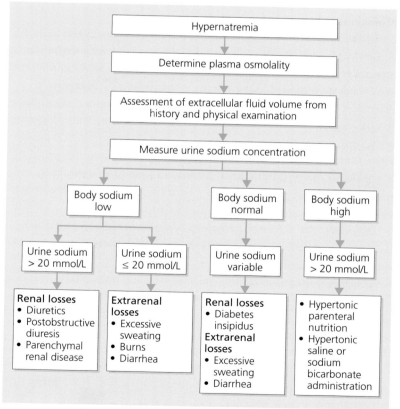

**Figure 2.1** Diagnostic approach to the causes of hypernatremia.

hypernatremia are treated with diuretics and free water given orally or parenterally (5% dextrose). Euvolemic hypernatremic patients can be treated with free water orally or 5% dextrose infusion. Too rapid correction is associated with brain edema, caused by the rapid movement of water into the brain, and seizures. In most circumstances, a correction rate of about 0.5 mmol/L/hour should suffice.

## Potassium disorders

Potassium is predominantly found intracellularly. Excretion of potassium is largely achieved by the kidneys, but also to a lesser extent by the colon. Transcellular shifts of potassium between the intracellular and extracellular compartments also occur.

**Hypokalemia** (plasma potassium ≤ 3.5 mmol/L) is one of the most common electrolyte abnormalities in hospitalized patients (Table 2.5).

*Clinical features* largely reflect alterations in membrane polarization, especially in cardiac and skeletal muscle. Changes in the electrocardiogram (ECG) include flattening of the T wave, depression of ST segments and a prominent U wave (Figure 2.2). Hypokalemia also increases predisposition to arrhythmias, particularly in patients with digoxin toxicity or those with acute coronary syndromes. The effects of hypokalemia on skeletal muscle range from weakness, tetany and fatigue to rhabdomyolosis. Severe hypokalemia (plasma potassium < 2.0 mmol/L) can lead to paralysis. Chronic hypokalemia can also cause a reduction in glomerular filtration rate (GFR), interstitial scarring and tubular atrophy.

*Diagnosis.* The differential diagnosis of the causes of hypokalemia is shown in Figure 2.3. Hypokalemia due to excessive loss is the most common cause; renal losses usually occur with the use of diuretics, metabolic acidosis and alkalosis. The most common transcellular shift occurs because of an abrupt increase in plasma catecholamines during an episode of intense stress, which activates the $\beta_2$-adrenergic receptor.

*Treatment* of hypokalemia depends on its severity and duration, and the underlying clinical context. Giving no treatment carries the risk of tachyarrhythmias, while aggressive treatment with potassium may result in hyperkalemia. Treatment is recommended for patients with a plasma potassium level below 3 mmol/L, regardless of the duration and the clinical context. In normal individuals, mild hypokalemia (plasma

TABLE 2.5

**Causes of hypo- and hyperkalemia**

| Hypokalemia | Hyperkalemia |
| --- | --- |
| **Reduced intake** | **Increased intake** |
| • Dietary deficiency (tea-and-toast diet) | • Potassium supplements |
| | • Medications (penicillin) |
| | • Endogenous sources |
| |   – rhabdomyolyis |
| |   – severe exercise |
| |   – intravascular hemolysis |
| **Transcellular shifts** | **Transcellular shifts** |
| • Catecholamines (β2-agonists) | • Non-selective β-blockers |
| • Insulin | • Hyperglycemia |
| • Alkalemia | • Digoxin intoxication |
| | • Acidosis |
| **Renal losses** | **Reduced renal losses** |
| • Renal tubular acidosis | • Acute kidney injury |
| • Diuretics | • Chronic kidney disease |
| • Bartter's syndrome | • Medications |
| • Magnesium deficiency |   – spironolactone, amiloride |
| |   – angiotensin-converting enzyme inhibitors or angiotensin-receptor blockers |
| |   – ciclosporin A |
| |   – triamterene |
| **Extrarenal losses** | |
| • Skin – excessive sweating | |
| • Gastrointestinal – diarrhea, fistulas | |
| • Vomiting and nasogastric drainage | |

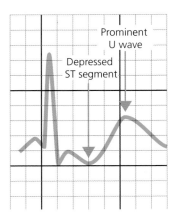

**Figure 2.2** Changes in the ECG associated with hypokalemia, including flattening of the T wave, depression of ST segments and a prominent U wave.

Labels in figure: Prominent U wave; Depressed ST segment

potassium 3.0–3.5 mmol/L), particularly if chronic, may not need treatment. On the other hand, even mild hypokalemia should be treated in patients receiving digoxin, individuals with structural or ischemic heart disease and patients with decompensated liver disease.

Oral therapy is preferable in chronic and/or mild hypokalemia. Intravenous potassium should be used cautiously (at a rate of < 10 mmol/hour), under cardiac monitoring and with follow-up measurements of plasma potassium.

**Hyperkalemia** (plasma potassium > 5.0 mmol/L) is common (see Table 2.5). Spurious hyperkalemia is not uncommon, and is usually the result of hemolysis caused by excessively tight or prolonged application of a tourniquet, underlying red-cell abnormalities or an extremely high platelet count.

The most common renal cause of hyperkalemia is chronic kidney disease (CKD), but this hyperkalemia usually only occurs when the GFR has fallen to less than 10 mL/minute. Aldosterone deficiency may be superimposed on CKD and is often acquired, for example with the use of drugs such as angiotensin-converting enzyme (ACE) inhibitors and non-steroidal anti-inflammatory drugs (NSAIDs).

*Clinical features.* The clinical effects of hyperkalemia particularly affect the heart. ECG features include peaking or tenting of T waves, flattening of the P wave, prolongation of the PR interval and widening of the QRS complex (Figure 2.4). Ventricular fibrillation is the most severe consequence. Hyponatremic and hypocalcemic patients appear most

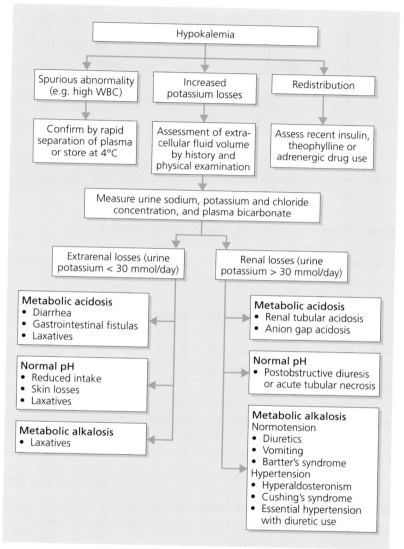

**Figure 2.3** Diagnosis of cause of hypokalemia. WBC, white blood cell.

vulnerable. Other manifestations include tingling, paresthesias, weakness and flaccid paralysis, nausea, vomiting and abdominal pain.

*Diagnosis.* The key differential diagnosis is spurious hyperkalemia from hemolysis, often during the phlebotomy.

25

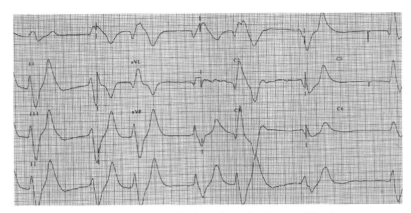

**Figure 2.4** Hyperkalemia causes slowing of conduction, resulting in an increased PR interval, shortening of the QT interval and peaked T waves on the ECG. With more severe hyperkalemia (> 6.5 mEq/L), the QRS interval widens further and the P wave disappears. Finally, the QRS complex degenerates into a sinusoidal pattern, and ventricular fibrillation or asystole ensues.

*Treatment* of hyperkalemia depends on its severity and duration, and the clinical context. The presence of ECG changes and/or an absolute plasma potassium level above 6.5 mmol/L is an emergency. Immediate treatment with intravenous calcium chloride or calcium gluconate as a cardioprotective agent should be given, followed by steps to reduce the plasma potassium level either by inducing a transcellular shift of potassium from the extracellular to intracellular compartment (insulin/dextrose, salbutamol and treatment of acidosis if present) or by increasing potassium excretion (loop diuretics, sodium polystyrene or calcium resonium, or dialysis).

## Disorders of calcium metabolism

The kidneys, intestine, bone and several hormones are involved in maintaining calcium balance.

**Hypocalcemia.** Since 70% of serum calcium is bound to albumin, the most common cause of hypocalcemia is a low plasma albumin concentration. This is false or spurious hypocalcemia (Table 2.6).

*Clinical features.* The most common clinical manifestations of hypocalcemia are neuromuscular (e.g. tetany, seizures), ECG abnormalities

TABLE 2.6

**Causes of hypo- and hypercalcemia**

| Hypocalcemia | Hypercalcemia |
|---|---|
| • Primary hypoparathyroidism<br> – idiopathic<br> – postsurgical<br>• Pseudohypoparathyroidism<br>• Acute pancreatitis<br>• Hypocalcemia associated with malignancy<br>• Toxic shock syndrome<br>• Vitamin D deficiency<br> – malabsorption<br> – diet<br> – chronic kidney disease<br> – chronic hepatic disease<br> – antiseizure therapy | • Primary hyperparathyroidism<br>• Hypercalcemia of malignancy<br>• Thyrotoxicosis<br>• Sarcoidosis<br>• Tuberculosis<br>• Vitamin D intoxication<br>• Milk-alkali syndrome<br>• Immobilization<br>• Paget's disease<br>• Chronic kidney disease (when treated for associated bone disease or with tertiary hyperparathyroidism) |

(e.g. prolongation of the QTc and ST intervals, T wave peaking, T wave inversion) and psychiatric (e.g. confusion, depression, irritability). The classic clinical signs are Chvostek's and Trousseau's signs. Chvostek's sign is an abnormal reaction to tapping the facial nerve immediately as it exits the auditory canal, which represents momentary contraction of facial muscles on the same side as the stimulation (typically a twitch of the nose or lips); however, Chvostek's sign may be positive in 10% of normal individuals. Trousseau's sign involves pumping a blood pressure cuff 3 mmHg above the systolic blood pressure and maintaining it for 10 minutes. A positive Trousseau's sign is present when the muscles of the hand and forearm spasmodically contract, including adduction of the fingers.

*Diagnosis* always requires measurement of calcium corrected for serum albumin.

*Treatment.* In general, patients with a calcium level corrected to below 1.75 mmol/L (7 mg/dL) or those with tetany, seizures and/or ECG abnormalities should be treated. Patients who are asymptomatic with a chronically low calcium level can be treated with oral calcium salts, vitamin D and the use of a thiazide to reduce renal excretion of calcium; calcium carbonate contains more elemental calcium than other salts. Patients with symptomatic and severe hypocalcemia must be given intravenous calcium with a bolus of calcium gluconate (10 mL of 10% calcium gluconate), under cardiac monitoring. Calcium gluconate is preferable to calcium chloride, because calcium chloride can cause tissue necrosis if accidentally extravasated.

**Hypercalcemia.** The most common cause of hypercalcemia among hospitalized patients is an underlying malignancy, whereas in a community outpatient setting the most common cause is primary hyperparathyroidism (see Table 2.6).

*Clinical features.* Neurological features are usually the earliest manifestations of hypercalcemia, and gastrointestinal symptoms are often disabling (Table 2.7).

*Diagnosis.* All patients require a careful search for underlying malignancy and measurement of parathyroid hormone (PTH) level. In primary hyperparathyroidism the PTH is not suppressed by the raised calcium. Almost all other causes of hypercalcemia have a low or undetectable PTH level.

*Treatment.* Symptomatic patients with a serum calcium level of 3.25 mmol/L (13 mg/dL) or more require urgent treatment, initially hydration with normal saline and diuretic therapy with furosemide. For patients with hypercalcemia secondary to a neoplasm, additional plicamycin (mithramycin), corticosteroids or bisphosphonates should be considered (cautiously in kidney failure). Because bisphosphonates take 2–3 days to achieve maximum effect, calcitonin can be considered as a short-term therapy (effective within about 12 hours). Corticosteroids are commonly used for hematologic malignancies and are usually very effective.

## Acid–base disorders

The normal range of the arterial pH is 7.36–7.44. Homeostatic mechanisms include systemic buffering of acid by both the circulation and bone, and the involvement of the respiratory and renal systems. Circulating and intracellular buffers quickly neutralize an acid load;

TABLE 2.7

**Clinical manifestations of hypercalcemia**

**Neurological**
- Headache
- Muscle weakness
- Hypotonia
- Stupor
- Confusion
- Coma

**Psychiatric**
- Depression
- Irritability
- Hallucinations

**Gastrointestinal**
- Nausea
- Vomiting
- Constipation
- Pancreatitis

**Cardiovascular**
- Electrocardiographic changes

**Renal**
- Polyuria
- Reduced glomerular filtration rate

however, the capacity of these buffering systems is soon exhausted in the absence of mechanisms to excrete acid. The two major organs that eliminate acid are the lungs and the kidneys. Acid is eliminated by the lungs in the form of carbon dioxide. The kidneys contribute by excreting acid as well as reclaiming bicarbonate.

**Assessment of acid–base status.** The first step in the evaluation of an acid–base problem is to measure serum electrolytes and arterial blood gases. After determining whether the patient has a metabolic/respiratory acidosis/alkalosis, the appropriateness of the secondary (or compensatory) physiological response should be assessed. In metabolic acidosis, calculation of the anion gap (i.e. serum sodium plus potassium minus serum chloride and bicarbonate) is very useful.

**Metabolic acidosis** is characterized by a primary decrease in the serum bicarbonate concentration. This occurs because of depletion or consumption of bicarbonate to buffer exogenous or endogenous generation of acid. Metabolic acidosis can be subdivided into that with an elevated anion gap and that with a normal anion gap (Table 2.8).

TABLE 2.8

**Causes of metabolic acidosis**

**Normal anion gap\***
- Gastrointestinal
  - diarrhea
  - ureteroileostomy
- Renal
  - renal tubular acidosis
  - aldosterone deficiency (hyporeninemic hypoaldosteronism)
- Drugs
  - ammonium chloride
  - lysine or arginine hydrochloride

**Elevated anion gap\***
- Diabetic ketoacidosis
- Alcoholic ketoacidosis
- Starvation ketoacidosis
- Lactic acidosis
- Ingestion of toxins (methanol, ethylene glycol, salicylates, paraldehyde)
- Chronic kidney disease

\*Anion gap = serum $(Na^+ + K^+) - (Cl^- + HCO_3^-)$.

In proximal renal tubular acidosis, the primary defect is impaired reabsorption of bicarbonate by the proximal tubule. It is often associated with defective phosphate, glucose, urate and amino acid reabsorption. In distal renal tubular acidosis, the primary defect is an inability to acidify the urine maximally. Type 4 renal tubular acidosis is characterized by impaired urinary acidification caused by hypoaldosteronism. Lactic acidosis is often observed in critically ill hospitalized patients and reflects decreased tissue oxygenation.

The treatment of metabolic acidosis depends on the underlying cause and the severity of manifestations. In general, a pH of below 7.1, especially if it is associated with hemodynamic instability, should be treated by parenteral administration of sodium bicarbonate. In patients with chronic metabolic acidosis, such as a patient with a renal tubular acidosis, oral repletion with sodium bicarbonate is sufficient.

**Metabolic alkalosis** is characterized by a primary increase in the serum bicarbonate concentration. The most common causes are vomiting, diuretics and potassium depletion. The clinical features include muscle spasms, confusion, Chvostek's or Trousseau's signs (see page 27), lethargy, seizures, coma and ventilatory depression.

After confirming the presence of metabolic alkalosis, the underlying cause should be identified together with the factors responsible for maintaining the alkalosis, especially extracellular volume depletion. The treatment of a metabolic alkalosis depends on identifying and remedying the underlying cause.

**Respiratory acidosis and alkalosis** are a consequence of primary abnormalities in the pulmonary mechanisms that maintain arterial pH. Respiratory acidosis results from impairment in the rate of alveolar ventilation. Acute respiratory acidosis is observed in situations in which there is a sudden depression of the medullary respiratory center, with paralysis of the muscles required for ventilation, or in airway obstruction. Chronic respiratory acidosis is observed in individuals with chronic airway disease.

Respiratory alkalosis occurs when hyperventilation reduces the arterial partial pressure of carbon dioxide and increases arterial pH. Acute respiratory alkalosis occurs most commonly as a result of the hyperventilation syndrome. It is characterized by lightheadedness, circumoral numbness and paresthesias; tetany may also occur.

## Key points – electrolyte disturbances and acid–base disorders

- Electrolyte disturbances are very common and often iatrogenic.
- All electrolye disturbances require an accurate assessment of fluid balance.
- Intake and excretion of solutes, and drugs, must be considered when trying to identify causes.
- Correction should generally be cautious.

## Key references

Adrogué HJ, Madias NE. Hypernatremia. *N Engl J Med* 2000;342:1493–9.

Adrogué HJ, Madias NE. Hyponatremia. *N Engl J Med* 2000;342:1581–9.

Ellison DH, Berl T. Clinical practice. The syndrome of inappropriate antidiuresis. *N Engl J Med* 2007;356:2064–72.

Kraut JA, Madias NE. Metabolic acidosis: pathophysiology, diagnosis and management. *Nat Rev Nephrol* 2010;6:274–85.

Kraut JA, Madias NE. Approach to patients with acid-base disorders. *Respir Care* 2001;46:392–403.

Nyirenda MJ, Tang JI, Padfield PL, Seckl JR. Hyperkalaemia. *BMJ* 2009;339:b4114.

Schaefer TJ, Wolford RW. Disorders of potassium. *Emerg Med Clin North Am* 2005;23:723–47,viii-ix.

# 3  Acute kidney injury

The term acute kidney injury (AKI) describes a sudden reduction in glomerular filtration rate (GFR), within days or weeks, resulting in the accumulation of fluid and nitrogenous waste products usually excreted by the kidneys.

AKI is seen in up to 5% of hospital patients, and is far more common in the elderly. Pregnancy can also cause AKI (Table 3.1), and renal disease can present for the first time during pregnancy. Pregnant women should be investigated as usual; kidney biopsy, if indicated, is safe.

The incidence of severe AKI (serum creatinine > 5.7 mg/dL [500 µmol/L]) is about 140/million/year. AKI may result from poor perfusion of the kidneys (prerenal), intrinsic renal disease or urinary tract obstruction (postrenal). In general, prerenal AKI will recover rapidly once kidney perfusion is re-established. However, reversible prerenal AKI overlaps with, and may lead to, established AKI owing to acute tubular necrosis (ATN). In ATN, the degree of tubular damage is such that kidney recovery is often delayed for 2 weeks or longer. ATN is by far the most common cause of AKI, and is often seen in postoperative patients in a hospital setting, and in those with severe infections or multisystem disease (Table 3.2).

TABLE 3.1

**Causes of acute kidney injury in pregnancy**

- Hemorrhage
- Hyperemesis
- Abruption
- Pre-eclampsia
- Hemolytic uremic syndrome
- Pyelonephritis
- Acute fatty liver of pregnancy
- Sepsis (including septic abortion)
- Acute hydronephrosis
- Trauma (e.g. damage to ureter during surgery)

TABLE 3.2

**Causes of acute kidney injury**

Prerenal

- Volume depletion (e.g. severe vomiting or diarrhea, burns, inappropriate diuretics)
- Hypotension (e.g. trauma, gastrointestinal hemorrhage)
- Cardiovascular (e.g. severe cardiac failure, arrhythmias)
- Drugs affecting kidney perfusion (e.g. NSAIDs, contrast media, ciclosporin, ACE inhibitors)
- Hepatorenal syndrome

Intrinsic AKI

- Acute tubular necrosis following prolonged ischemia
- Nephrotoxins (e.g. aminoglycosides, myoglobin, cisplatin, heavy metals, light chains in myeloma kidney)
- Acute interstitial nephritis due to drugs, infection or autoimmune diseases
- Glomerular damage (e.g. crescentic glomerulonephritis, vasculitis, hemolytic uremic syndrome)
- Vascular damage (e.g. renal artery occlusion, renal vein thrombosis, cholesterol emboli, scleroderma renal crisis, malignant hypertension)

Postrenal

- Ureteric obstruction (e.g. renal calculi, tumors, blood clots, retroperitoneal fibrosis)
- Bladder outlet obstruction (e.g. prostatic hypertrophy, bladder carcinoma)

ACE, angiotensin-converting enzyme; AKI, acute kidney injury; NSAID, non-steroidal anti-inflammatory drug.

## Important questions

**Is it truly prerenal AKI?** It is important to establish whether patients with poor kidney perfusion and accumulation of toxic metabolites have true prerenal AKI or whether they have established ATN. Urinary biochemistry may be helpful, since most patients with immediately reversible prerenal failure have a low urinary sodium concentration (< 20 mmol/L) and a high urine:plasma osmolality ratio (> 1.5). In practice, the management of patients will always include measures to increase kidney perfusion, so the key issue is whether or not kidney function shows a rapid response to intravenous fluid resuscitation.

**Were the kidneys previously normal?** It is important to establish whether acute uremia is due to AKI in previously normal kidneys, or whether it represents a rapid decline against a background of chronic kidney disease (CKD), i.e. acute on chronic kidney failure. The history and examination will provide clues, but renal ultrasonography will provide the most important information. In acute on chronic kidney failure, renal abnormalities, such as small kidneys in chronic glomerulonephritis or large cystic kidneys in adult polycystic kidney disease, will almost always be present. It is necessary to decide whether the acute uremic episode represents the natural history of these diseases, or whether exacerbating factors that may be reversible are responsible.

**Is an obstruction present?** If obstruction could be the cause of AKI, kidney function may improve rapidly once the obstruction is relieved. This should be revealed by renal ultrasonography.

**Is intrinsic renal disease, requiring urgent therapy, present?** Tubulointerstitial nephritis or glomerulonephritis may be suggested by abnormal findings on urine microscopy (e.g. hematuria, proteinuria, red-cell casts) (see Chapter 1).

**Is acute vascular occlusion present?** Possible occlusion should be assessed by Doppler ultrasonography of the renal artery and veins. If it is strongly suspected, more accurate imaging (for example, using magnetic resonance angiography) should be performed.

## Intrinsic renal disease

Established AKI is most often due to ATN. The most common cause of ATN is prolonged renal ischemia due to reduced kidney perfusion, which may be a result of volume depletion, septicemia, cardiac failure or renal artery obstruction. Tubular damage is often caused by exogenous toxins, such as non-steroidal anti-inflammatory drugs (NSAIDs), heavy metals and contrast agents. Endogenous tubular toxins, such as myoglobin (in rhabdomyolysis), hemoglobin (in hemolysis) or immunoglobulin light chains (in myeloma), are also important causes. It is essential to look for hematuria, urinary casts and proteinuria, which suggest a diagnosis of glomerulonephritis or tubulointerstitial nephritis. In these circumstances, kidney biopsy may be indicated. When the cause of AKI is unclear, a number of blood tests may be helpful (Table 3.3).

## Postrenal acute kidney injury

Postrenal AKI is usually the result of obstruction of the lower urinary tract by calculi, tumors or prostatic hypertrophy. In most cases (but not all), lower tract obstruction will lead to dilatation of the renal pelvis, which is visible on ultrasonography. AKI due to obstruction generally resolves once it is relieved by placement of a bladder catheter or percutaneous nephrostomy. Prolonged obstruction may lead to irreversible kidney damage. Less commonly, intrarenal obstruction occurs as a result of deposition of crystals in the tubules (e.g. oxalate in ethylene glycol poisoning).

TABLE 3.3

**Blood tests in acute kidney injury**

| Test | Diagnosis |
|------|-----------|
| Creatine kinase | Rhabdomyolysis |
| Eosinophilia | Acute interstitial nephritis<br>Cholesterol emboli |
| Anti-DNA antibodies | SLE |
| Low complement levels | SLE<br>Cryoglobulinemia<br>Cholesterol emboli |
| Cryoglobulins | Cryoglobulinemia |
| Antineutrophil cytoplasm antibodies | Systemic vasculitis |
| Anti-GBM antibodies | Goodpasture's syndrome |
| Serum electrophoresis (paraprotein) | Multiple myeloma |

GBM, glomerular basement membrane; SLE, systemic lupus erythematosus.

TABLE 3.4

**Management of acute kidney injury**

- Accurate control of fluid balance (avoid volume overload or depletion)
- Potassium restriction
- Daily measurement of serum electrolytes
- Nutritional support
- Careful drug dosing
- Avoidance of nephrotoxic drugs
- Specific treatment of underlying intrinsic renal disease where appropriate
- Dialysis or hemofiltration

## Management

Management of AKI includes the treatment of any underlying cause, general medical management of kidney failure and, if necessary, renal replacement therapy (dialysis). In prerenal failure, correction of volume depletion, using central venous pressure (CVP) monitoring when necessary, should result in rapid recovery of kidney function (Table 3.4). However, once ATN has developed, and in other causes of AKI, the patient will often be oliguric for several days or weeks.

Patients with ATN lose the ability both to concentrate and dilute the urine, and will pass a constant volume with inappropriate osmolality. Accurate measurement of urine output is essential to prevent volume overload or depletion. Most patients are oliguric and, in general, should be provided with a volume of fluid equal to the output on the previous day, plus at least an extra 500 mL if pyrexia is present. The situation may change rapidly and requires frequent clinical assessment together with CVP monitoring and measurement of body weight. Although diuretics do not alter the course or outcome of AKI, high-dose diuretics may convert oliguric AKI to non-oliguric AKI, which is worthwhile if dialysis is not readily available. There is no evidence in favor of using low-dose dopamine infusions; indeed, there is good evidence of a lack of benefit.

**Potassium and sodium levels.** Potassium restriction is nearly always necessary and is typically limited to less than 50 mmol/day. In the acute situation, hyperkalemia may be managed with dextrose/insulin infusions and administration of calcium gluconate. In the slightly longer term, potassium-binding resins can be used if dialysis is not immediately available. Sodium intake should be restricted to about 80 mmol/day, depending on losses. Serum potassium and sodium concentrations should be assessed daily. Acidosis may be limited by protein restriction, though a daily intake of at least approximately 1 g of high-quality protein per kilogram of body weight is necessary to maintain adequate nutrition. Sodium bicarbonate may be used to treat acidosis, but has the potential disadvantage that it may worsen sodium overload.

**Drug modification.** As many of the drugs prescribed for patients with AKI are excreted via the kidney, doses must be adjusted and drug levels monitored accordingly. Nephrotoxic drugs, such as NSAIDs and aminoglycosides, should be avoided.

As gastrointestinal hemorrhage is another potential cause of morbidity in AKI, prophylactic treatment to reduce acid secretion is generally indicated.

**Infection control.** Patients with kidney failure are susceptible to infection, so it is important to take great care of intravenous lines, to perform regular cultures of body fluids and to use antibiotics early.

**Nutrition.** It is important to maintain adequate nutrition, preferably via the enteral route, but using parenteral nutrition if necessary.

**Dialysis** is indicated to treat the clinical consequences of uremia and to control electrolyte, acid–base and fluid balance. In oliguric or anuric patients, the fluid intake required for feeding generally means that dialysis will be necessary (Table 3.5). Peritoneal dialysis is usually only performed when hemodialysis is unavailable. In patients who are hemodynamically unstable, particularly those in intensive care, continuous dialysis techniques (e.g. hemodiafiltration) are better tolerated than intermittent hemodialysis and allow more effective control of fluid balance.

## Specific treatments
Acute renal artery thrombosis (of a single functioning kidney) may be treated surgically, or by angioplasty and stenting. In rhabdomyolysis with

TABLE 3.5

**Indications for dialysis in acute kidney injury**

- Presence of clinical features of uremia (e.g. pericarditis, encephalopathy)
- Fluid retention leading to pulmonary edema
- Severe hyperkalemia unresponsive to medical management
- Acidosis that cannot be controlled by sodium bicarbonate
- Biochemical results indicating severe kidney failure (urea > 30 mmol/L [84 mg/dL], creatinine > 500 µmol/L [5.7 mg/dL]) and the presence of uremia (see Chapter 4)

myoglobulinuria, alkaline diuresis may prevent the development of severe kidney failure, but must be undertaken with care in oliguric patients. Acute tubulointerstitial nephritis may respond to a short course of high-dose corticosteroids, though no controlled trials have been undertaken to support this approach. AKI due to crescentic glomerulonephritis may respond to treatment with prednisolone and cyclophosphamide, together with the addition of plasma exchange (see Chapter 6). Hemolytic uremic syndrome (HUS) may respond to plasma exchange with fresh frozen plasma.

## Outcome

Most patients with ATN should recover kidney function, provided that they survive the underlying illness. However, increasingly it is being recognized that AKI is a risk factor for the subsequent development of CKD. Similarly, most patients will recover from acute interstitial nephritis. Recovery from crescentic glomerulonephritis is more variable; patients usually recover if treated early, but are likely to remain dependent on dialysis if treated late or inadequately.

Survival in AKI depends on the cause, and mortality remains high (40–80%) in patients with multiple organ failure. Death is likely if AKI is associated with failure of more than three other organ systems. In patients acquiring AKI in the community, however, mortality is much lower (10–30%).

**Key points – acute kidney injury**

- Acute kidney injury (AKI) is common and often reversible if diagnosed promptly.
- Recognition and management of volume depletion or overload is crucial in the early management of AKI.
- Patients require frequent re-assessment and measurement of physiological parameters (including urine output), and daily measurement of serum electrolytes.
- Drug doses often need to be modified.
- Acute tubular necrosis has no specific treatment other than volume control, and there is no benefit in the routine use of dopamine or furosemide.
- AKI is a risk factor for the subsequent development of chronic kidney disease.

**Key references**

Bagshaw SM, Wald R. Acute kidney injury in 2010: advances in diagnosis and estimating disease prognosis. *Nat Rev Nephrol* 2011;7:70–1.

Kinsey GR, Okusa MD. Pathogenesis of acute kidney injury: foundation for clinical practice. *Am J Kidney Dis* 2011;58:291–301.

Murugan R, Kellum JA. Acute kidney injury: what's the prognosis? *Nat Rev Nephrol* 2011;7:209–17.

Ricci Z, Cruz DN, Ronco C. Classification and staging of acute kidney injury: beyond the RIFLE and AKIN criteria. *Nat Rev Nephrol* 2011;7:201–8.

Sharfuddin AA, Molitoris BA. Pathophysiology of ischemic acute kidney injury. *Nat Rev Nephrol* 2011;7:189–200.

Chronic kidney disease (CKD) is common and underrecognized. It can be defined as kidney damage present for at least 3 months, with either structural or functional abnormalities of the kidney with or without decreased glomerular filtration rate (GFR). In the early stages of CKD, evidence of kidney damage (e.g. proteinuria, cysts, biopsy changes) may be seen in the presence of a normal GFR (> 60 mL/minute/1.73 m$^2$), while the later stages are characterized by greater functional impairment, with the GFR falling to below 60 mL/minute/1.73 m$^2$ (Table 4.1).

## Epidemiology

Approximately 11% of people in the USA (20 million) are estimated to have CKD stages 1–4, which far exceeds the 300 000 patients receiving hemodialysis. In the UK, 9% of the population (approximately 2 million individuals) have CKD stages 1–4 with about 20 000 patients on dialysis. This is particularly important, because much of the damage caused by CKD occurs early, when interventions may slow progressive kidney

TABLE 4.1

**Definition and stages of chronic kidney disease***

| GFR (mL/minute/1.73 m$^2$) | Disease stage | Comments |
|---|---|---|
| > 90 | 1 | Normal, if there is no kidney damage by any criterion |
| 60–89 | 2 | May be normal for age; represents decreased GFR only, if there is no kidney damage |
| 30–59 | 3 | Always abnormal |
| 15–29 | 4 | Always abnormal |
| < 15 or dialysis | 5 | End-stage renal failure |

*Modified from the National Kidney Foundation (USA) Kidney Disease Outcomes Quality Initiative (K/DOQI) guidelines, 2002. GFR, glomerular filtration rate.

damage, prevent left ventricular hypertrophy, minimize vascular disease and improve quality of life.

The incidence of CKD leading to dialysis varies worldwide; the number of patients per million population starting dialysis each year is 300 in the USA compared with 230 in Japan and 110 in the UK. The prevalence of end-stage kidney disease (ESKD) also varies; in the USA, 1 in 1000 of the population are receiving treatment for ESKD (dialysis or transplantation) and, overall, the number of patients per million population is 1131 compared with 1397 in Japan, 690 in Canada, 634 in France, 530 in Australia, 498 in the UK and 223 in Poland. Reasons for this wide variation include both patient factors (e.g. the prevalence of diabetes) and external factors (e.g. the availability of dialysis and the number of nephrologists).

The three most important causes of CKD are diabetes, glomerulonephritis and hypertension (and other vascular disease), but the primary cause does vary geographically (Figure 4.1). However, kidney failure resulting from diabetes and hypertension is potentially preventable (see Chapter 5), and many causes of glomerulonephritis can be treated if diagnosed at an early stage (see Chapter 6). The incidence of CKD due to hypertension may be overestimated in countries with a conservative approach to renal biopsy.

## Clinical features

CKD usually presents with non-specific symptoms caused by kidney failure and the underlying disease, or is discovered by chance following a routine blood or urine test. Specific symptoms usually develop only in severe kidney failure. The presence of one or more of these symptoms (and signs) are collectively referred to as uremia. The most common symptoms in late kidney failure include anorexia, nausea, vomiting, fatigue, weakness, pruritus, edema, lethargy, dyspnea, insomnia, muscle cramps, pulmonary edema, nocturia, polyuria and headache. Sexual dysfunction is rarely reported voluntarily, but is common. Hiccups, pericarditis, coma and seizures are seldom seen except in developing countries when kidney disease presents very late.

Signs of CKD include skin pigmentation or excoriation, anemia, hypertension, postural hypotension, edema, left ventricular hypertrophy, peripheral vascular disease, lung crackles, pleural effusions, peripheral neuropathy and urine abnormalities (presence of blood or protein).

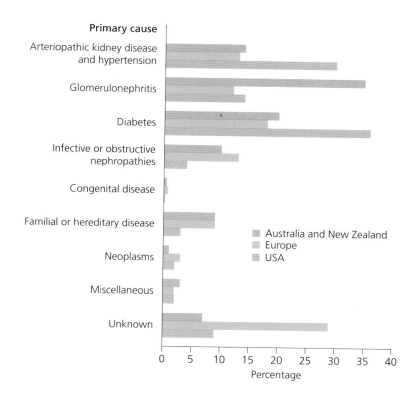

**Figure 4.1** Causes of end-stage kidney disease (data from renal registries).

## Diagnosis

Recognition of abnormal kidney function is the key to the diagnosis of CKD. However, blood urea nitrogen (BUN or serum urea) is an extremely poor marker of kidney function, because it varies significantly with hydration status and diet, it is not produced constantly and it is reabsorbed by the kidney. Historically, serum creatinine has been used, but this also has significant limitations, particularly the fact that the level can remain within the normal range despite the loss of over 50% of kidney function. A 'gold-standard' measurement is an isotopic glomerular filtration rate (GFR), but this is expensive and not available in community settings. It is now clear that calculated GFR using a formula based on serum creatinine is preferred, and can be a valid, reliable, repeatable and reasonably accurate measure of true GFR in patients with renal impairment (see Table 1.4, page 13). Measurement of serum cystatin C is also a reliable marker of GFR, but this test is not yet widely available.

## Management

CKD is generally a progressive disease (Figure 4.2), though the rate of decline in kidney function varies between patients. In the last decade, it has become clear that, regardless of the underlying cause of the kidney disease, the factors that will determine the likelihood of progression to ESKD are:

- the level of albuminuria
- the initial degree of renal impairment
- blood pressure.

Treatments aimed at reducing albuminuria and vigorously controlling blood pressure have been shown to slow or even halt the decline in kidney function and to reduce the vascular complications, which are the leading cause of death in CKD. Even a relatively small change in the progression of kidney failure has enormous implications both for the individual patient (quality of life declines significantly once dialysis is needed) and for governments or insurers (dialysis is expensive and even a small delay before it is necessary saves millions of dollars a year).

The management of CKD is summarized in Tables 4.2 and 4.3. Blood pressure targets are extremely low and some drugs are undoubtedly more beneficial than others (e.g. angiotensin-converting enzyme [ACE]

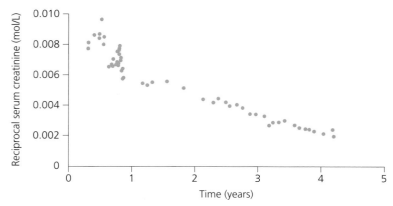

**Figure 4.2** Steady decline in kidney function over time as shown by the reciprocal serum creatinine plot.

TABLE 4.2

**Clinical approach in chronic kidney disease\***

| | GFR (mL/minute/1.73 m²) | Management |
|---|---|---|
| **Stage 1** | | |
| Kidney damage with normal GFR | ≥ 90 | Diagnose and treat underlying cause |
| | | Treat comorbid condition |
| | | Slow progression by controlling blood pressure and reducing proteinuria |
| | | Reduce cardiovascular risk |
| **Stage 2** | | |
| Kidney damage with mild decrease in GFR | 60–89 | As for stage 1 and estimate progression |
| **Stage 3** | | |
| Moderate decrease in GFR | 30–59 | Prevent and treat complications |
| **Stage 4** | | |
| Severe reduction in GFR | 15–29 | Prepare for renal replacement therapy (dialysis or transplantation) |
| **Stage 5** | | |
| Kidney failure | < 15 (or dialysis) | Renal replacement therapy |

\*Modified from the National Kidney Foundation (USA) Kidney Disease Outcomes Quality Initiative (K/DOQI) guidelines, 2002. GFR, glomerular filtration rate.

inhibitors in patients with albuminuria), though in reality all classes of drug need to be used for blood-pressure control, and most patients will require at least three or four drugs. Evidence suggests that for patients with CKD and albuminuria the target blood pressure should be between 125/75 mmHg and 130/80 mmHg, whereas in patients with CKD but no albuminuria, aiming for a blood pressure of less than 140/90 mmHg is recommended. Patients with diabetes undoubtedly benefit from renin-angiotensin blockade with either an ACE inhibitor or an angiotensin-

TABLE 4.3

## Management of chronic kidney disease

### Blood pressure

- Aim for < 130/80 mmHg in patients with albuminuria and < 140/90 mmHg in patients without albuminuria
- Use ACE inhibitors in all patients if tolerated and if renal artery stenosis is not present to slow disease progression (independent of their blood-pressure-lowering effect)

### Albuminuria

- Reduce albuminuria as much as possible; ACE inhibitors and ARBs are particularly effective, but diltiazem, verapamil and thiazide diuretics can also be used

### Conventional cardiovascular risk factors

- Stop smoking
- Eat a low-salt diet
- Take regular exercise
- Treat hypercholesterolemia, if present, with a statin
- (No evidence of benefit of folic acid in hyperhomocysteinemia)

### Acidosis*

- Treat with sodium bicarbonate, but can cause fluid overload and worsen hypertension

### Hyperphosphatemia†

- Treat with dietary restriction and phosphate binders

### Malnutrition

- Must be avoided, although protein restriction can slow progression

*May hasten CKD progression, and contribute to bone disease and muscle breakdown.
†Occurs late in CKD (usually stage 4 or 5).
ACE, angiotensin-converting enzyme; ARB, angiotensin-receptor blocker; CKD, chronic kidney disease.

receptor blocker (ARB). Combining both an ACE inhibitor and an ARB is no longer recommended for most patients. For patients on dialysis, the most important factor in controlling blood pressure is to control salt (and water) intake and body fluid volume. A full discussion of hypertension and kidney disease can be found in Chapter 5.

Evidence shows that early referral to a nephrologist reduces morbidity and early mortality in ESKD. Plans for renal replacement therapy when it becomes necessary require careful consideration. Patients being considered for predialysis transplantation, from either a living donor or a cadaver, require a full assessment of their suitability for the procedure. Patients need to be educated about the methods of dialysis (and conservative care), preservation of forearm veins and, if opting for hemodialysis, early formation of an arteriovenous fistula to avoid the need for intravenous dialysis catheters. Patients should also be vaccinated against hepatitis B early in CKD, when the immune response is better preserved.

## Complications

CKD leads to a variety of complications, which can all cause considerable morbidity (Table 4.4). One of the major aims of care in patients with CKD is to minimize these complications, even if the underlying renal disease cannot be treated. Many complications are common to both CKD and patients established on dialysis. Further investigations to identify complications of renal disease and to establish the underlying cause are summarized in Table 4.5.

**Anemia** is universal in ESKD and is largely due to a relative lack of erythropoietin. It usually develops when the GFR falls below 35 mL/minute and worsens as the GFR declines further. It is not solely due to erythropoietin deficiency; red-cell survival is shortened in uremia, iron deficiency is common, and vitamin $B_{12}$ and folate deficiencies also occur. Furthermore, patients may have a hemoglobinopathy or hemolysis, and hyperparathyroidism inhibits red-cell production. There is a strong association between anemia and risk of death in ESKD, and an association with increasing cardiovascular morbidity and mortality in CKD. However, several randomized trials have failed to demonstrate that correcting anemia leads to an improvement in quality of life, reduction in cardiovascular events or mortality.

TABLE 4.4

**Complications of chronic kidney disease**

| Complication | Effect |
|---|---|
| Anemia | Left ventricular hypertrophy, fatigue, impaired cognitive functioning |
| Hypertension | Left ventricular hypertrophy, heart failure, stroke, cardiovascular disease |
| Calcium phosphate imbalance | Cardiovascular and cerebrovascular disease, vascular calcification, arthropathy, soft tissue calcification |
| Metabolic bone disease | Bone pain, fractures |
| Dialysis amyloid | Bone pain, arthropathy, carpal tunnel syndrome |
| Fluid overload | Pulmonary edema, hypertension |
| Malnutrition | Increased morbidity and mortality, infections, poor wound healing |

Investigations to exclude other causes of anemia in CKD patients should include blood film, red-cell indices, white cells and platelets, serum iron, ferritin and transferrin saturation, serum vitamin $B_{12}$ and red-cell folate. If no cause is found, erythropoietin deficiency is likely and replacement therapy can be considered. Current evidence suggests that in most patients there is no benefit in correcting mild anemia (hemoglobin 10–12 g/dL) and treatment with an erythropoietin-stimulating agent (ESA) is often unnecessary. The decision to treat patients with more severe anemia (hemoglobin < 10 g/dL) with an ESA should be individualized. Preventing blood transfusions, especially in patients who are candidates for kidney transplantation, is an acceptable reason for ESA treatment. Several ESAs (e.g. Eprex, Epogen, Procrit, NeoRecormon, Aranesp) are now approved and widely available, all of which are effective (but expensive). They are usually given one to three times per week by subcutaneous or intravenous injection. (Eprex is only given intravenously as it has been associated with immunologic toxicity.) Patients need replete iron stores in order to benefit from erythropoietin and therefore should usually be given iron intravenously.

TABLE 4.5

**Investigation of complications in chronic kidney disease**

| Investigation | Comment |
| --- | --- |
| Serum sodium | Usually normal, but may be low |
| Serum potassium | Raised, often with a precipitant, but usually controllable by diet |
| Serum bicarbonate | Low, may need treatment |
| Serum albumin | Low levels at start of dialysis strongly associated with poor prognosis. Reflects both inflammation and malnutrition |
| Serum calcium | May be normal, low or high |
| Serum phosphate | Usually high and leads to vascular calcification |
| Serum alkaline phosphatase | Raised when bone disease develops |
| Plasma glucose | To detect undiagnosed diabetes or assess diabetic control |
| Serum parathyroid hormone | Rises progressively with declining kidney function |
| Serum cholesterol and triglycerides | Dyslipidemia common, often with raised triglycerides |
| Hemoglobin | Low and falls with progressive kidney failure |
| Serum ferritin | Large iron stores needed to utilize prescribed erythropoietin |
| White cells and platelets | Usually normal |
| Clotting | Normal |
| HLA tissue typing | Performed as a prelude to transplantation |
| Hepatitis serology | Ensure not infected and vaccinate against hepatitis B |
| HIV serology | Performed before dialysis or transplantation |
| ECG and echocardiography | To detect left ventricular hypertrophy and ischemia, and to assess cardiac function |
| Renal ultrasound | To confirm diagnosis or exclude treatable acute kidney failure |

ECG, electrocardiogram; HIV, human immunodeficiency virus; HLA, human leukocyte antigen.

TABLE 4.6

**Risk factors for cardiovascular disease in chronic kidney disease**

| General risk factors | Risk factors unique to kidney failure |
| --- | --- |
| • Age | • Anemia |
| • Male sex | • Hyperparathyroidism |
| • Smoking | • Uremia |
| • Family history | • Hyperphosphatemia |
| • Thrombogenic factors | • Malnutrition |
| • Obesity | • Arteriovenous fistulas |
| | • Volume overload |

**Risk factors with increased prevalence in kidney failure**

- Hypertension
- Diabetes
- Physical inactivity
- Left ventricular hypertrophy
- Cholesterol
- Lipoprotein (a)
- Homocysteine

**Cardiovascular problems.** Cardiovascular disease is the most common cause of death in patients with CKD, and cardiovascular mortality is doubled in patients with a GFR below 70 mL/minute (i.e. quite moderate renal impairment).

The risk factors for cardiovascular disease in CKD are summarized in Table 4.6; the risks increase as kidney function deteriorates. The major cardiovascular outcomes include stroke, sudden death, arrhythmia, myocardial infarction, ischemic heart disease, cardiac arrest, hypertension, pericarditis, left ventricular hypertrophy and vascular calcification (Figure 4.3).

Treatment of hyperlipidemia (elevated low-density lipoprotein [LDL]) has been shown to reduce the risk of cardiovascular events and mortality. Table 4.7 provides guidelines for reducing the risk of cardiovascular complications.

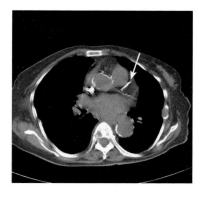

**Figure 4.3** CT scan showing coronary artery (white arrow) and aortic calcification (red arrow) in a patient with end-stage kidney disease.

TABLE 4.7

**Measures to reduce cardiovascular outcomes in chronic kidney disease**

| Risk factor | Target and/or treatment |
| --- | --- |
| Smoking | Smoking cessation |
| Hypertension | Reduce blood pressure to < 140/90 mmHg in patients without albuminuria and < 130/80 mmHg in patients with albuminuria |
| Diabetes | Reduce glycosylated hemoglobin to < 7.0% |
| Thrombogenic factors | ASA, 75 or 81 mg/day, unless contraindicated |
| Obesity | Appropriate dietary advice |
| Physical inactivity | Encourage exercise |
| Left ventricular hypertrophy | Control blood pressure |
| Cholesterol | Reduce to < 5.0 mmol/L |
| Lipoprotein (a) | No treatment available |
| Anemia | Hb to > 10 g/dL with iron and EPO |
| Hyperparathyroidism | Reduce PTH to < 2–9 times the upper limit of normal with vitamin D analogs or calcimimetics |
| Hyperphosphatemia | Reduce PO4 to < 2.0 mmol/L with PO4 binders |
| Uremia | Ensure dialysis adequate |
| Malnutrition | Improve nutrition as much as possible |

ASA, acetylsalicylic acid (aspirin); EPO, erythropoietin; Hb, hemoglobin; PO4, phosphate; PTH, parathyroid hormone.

In general, the management of cardiovascular disease is similar in patients with and without kidney disease. Care needs to be taken over drug dosing (e.g. avoiding long-acting β-blockers). Patients with CKD undergoing angiography should be protected from contrast nephropathy by hydration. Although thrombolysis and surgery can be safely carried out, surgery can cause hypotension, leading to acute deterioration in kidney function. Control of calcium and phosphate balance is recommended in later kidney failure to avoid vascular calcification and stiffening.

Hypertension can be both a cause and consequence of kidney disease, and uncontrolled hypertension is the most important factor contributing to the rate of progression of kidney damage, whatever the original cause (see Chapter 5). In addition to slowing or preventing the progression of CKD, tight blood pressure control also reduces overall cardiovascular outcomes and improves left ventricular hypertrophy.

**Metabolic bone disease.** A number of factors contribute to metabolic bone disease (Table 4.8). Furthermore, the complications of calcium and phosphate balance not only affect the skeleton, but are now known to contribute to vascular disease. Osteodystrophy develops at a relatively early stage of kidney failure, when the GFR falls below 30–40 mL/minute, and all patients with ESKD develop some manifestations of bone disease. The main underlying cause is decreased production of 1,25-dihydroxyvitamin D, which causes hypocalcemia and leads to increased secretion of parathyroid hormone (PTH) (Figure 4.4). Phosphate retention also begins relatively early and further stimulates PTH secretion. Hyperparathyroidism initially corrects the biochemical abnormalities by increasing phosphate excretion, stimulating vitamin D synthesis and increasing serum calcium levels, but at the expense of the skeleton, which can develop osteitis fibrosa. Independently, vitamin D deficiency can lead to osteomalacia.

Symptoms of metabolic bone disease include pruritus and bone and joint pain. Among the biochemical features are raised serum phosphate, raised serum PTH, and low or low-normal serum calcium. Calcium levels rise only after treatment with vitamin D analogs or calcium salts. Elevated levels of alkaline phosphatase are seen in established osteomalacia.

The aims of treatment include prevention of hyperphosphatemia, maintenance of normal serum calcium and inhibition of hyper-

TABLE 4.8

**Factors contributing to metabolic bone disease**

- Hyperparathyroidism
- Acidosis
- Low levels of vitamin D (in some patients)
- Suppressed parathyroid activity (after treatment)
- Aluminum accumulation (now rare)
- Osteoporosis in elderly patients
- Osteopenia caused by corticosteroids used to treat initial disease or for transplantation

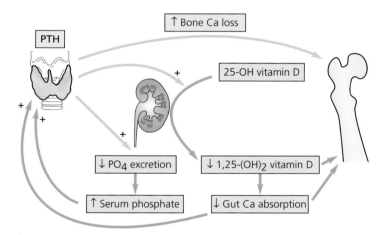

**Figure 4.4** In metabolic bone disease, decreased production of 1,25-dihydroxy-vitamin D stimulates parathyroid hormone (PTH) secretion, and causes hypocalcemia, further increasing secretion of PTH. Phosphate retention also stimulates PTH secretion. Bone disease is a consequence of both high PTH and low vitamin D levels.

parathyroidism. Patients need comprehensive advice about low-phosphate diets, and usually need to take phosphate binders with meals to reduce absorption of dietary phosphate. (Historically, aluminum salts were given, until it was recognized that aluminum itself caused neurological damage, anemia and bone disease.) Calcium salts have also been widely used, because they also treat hypocalcemia. However, there is evidence to suggest that the calcium absorbed in this way may contribute to vascular calcification and increased cardiovascular morbidity and mortality in ESKD. Non-calcium phosphate binders (sevelamer and lanthanum) are increasingly being used.

Vitamin D analogs can effectively suppress PTH, but sometimes at the price of encouraging hypercalcemia. Calcimimetic agents (cinacalcet) can also lower PTH levels without affecting serum calcium. Some patients require parathyroidectomy if all else fails.

**Dialysis amyloid** is a complication that affects all patients who have been on dialysis for over 20 years. It is caused by the accumulation of β2-microglobulin, which is deposited as amyloid in joints and bone. The initial manifestation is usually carpal tunnel syndrome, often about 7 years after the start of dialysis. Later, joint pains start in the shoulders and are worse at night, together with tenosynovitis of the finger flexors, destructive spondylarthropathy of the cervical spine and, occasionally, soft tissue accumulation. Radiographs may show bone cysts.

Dialysis amyloid can be treated only by kidney transplantation, and symptoms and signs may take years to abate; other treatments are palliative. It must, therefore, be prevented by using newer dialysis membranes and techniques (diafiltration) for hemodialysis, and longer hours of dialysis.

**Fluid overload, diet and nutrition.** Patients with ESKD are often almost anuric and must therefore watch their fluid intake carefully. This is particularly a problem for patients on hemodialysis. Fluid overload can lead to pulmonary edema, peripheral edema and hypertension. Some patients with CKD retain salt and water, and develop fluid overload requiring diuretics, while others lose salt and water, and become volume depleted, possibly requiring treatment with oral sodium bicarbonate.

Malnutrition is a particularly important problem in ESKD, and affects 40–50% of patients (Table 4.9). It is associated with an increased number of infections, muscle wasting, poor wound healing, and increased morbidity and mortality. The complexities of maintaining nutritional requirements in ESKD while limiting protein, salt, phosphate and fluid intake require the assistance of dietitians from an early stage in CKD.

TABLE 4.9

## Causes of malnutrition in end-stage kidney disease

### Factors increasing nutrient requirements

*Metabolic abnormalities*

- Altered amino acid and lipid metabolism
- Impaired glucose tolerance
- Hyperparathyroidism
- Metabolic acidosis
- Carnitine depletion
- Increased cytokine and leptin activity
- Uremia

*Concomitant disease*

- Cardiovascular disease
- Sepsis
- Inflammation

### Factors decreasing food intake

*Anorexia*

- Nausea
- Fatigue
- Taste changes
- Anemia
- Medications

*Gastrointestinal disturbances*

- Phosphate binders
- Hypoalbuminemia
- Antibiotics
- Uremic and diabetic gastroparesis

*Psychosocial and socioeconomic*

- Depression
- Anxiety
- Ignorance
- Loneliness
- Alcohol or drug abuse
- Poverty

Serum albumin is often used as an indication of nutritional state, but it must be remembered that it also falls in inflammatory conditions. A global evaluation of nutrition is much more useful, for example the subjective global assessment, which incorporates measures of dietary intake, comorbidity, functional capabilities and changes in body weight.

**Sexual, psychological and social complications.** Sexual dysfunction is extremely common in patients with CKD. Decreased libido, erectile dysfunction, amenorrhea and infertility may occur, often compounded by depression, anxiety and changes in body image.

Depression affects up to 60% of patients with ESKD and can manifest in a variety of ways, many of which can also be consequences of uremia. Treatment involves high-quality dialysis and psychological or pharmacological interventions as appropriate. The side effects of psychotropic drugs are often increased in kidney failure.

Many patients in ESKD also face changes in employment, social status, ability to obtain insurance and mortgages, and ability to travel. Social support is therefore immensely important and increases survival.

## The epidemic of chronic kidney disease

The incidence of CKD is relatively very high in some populations such as Indian-Asians, African-Americans and Afro-Caribbeans, Native Americans and Australian Aboriginals. Much of this CKD is due to type 2 diabetes and to hypertension, but there are also unknown causes of kidney failure. In developing countries an epidemic of CKD has begun, often associated with a westernized (i.e. degraded) diet and an increase in population obesity and type 2 diabetes. Unless the rise is halted, or the disease properly treated, we may expect a huge increase in the potential need for renal replacement therapies and in death in developing countries that cannot afford dialysis.

---

### Key points – chronic kidney disease

- Chronic kidney disease is very common, especially the early stages.
- Early interventions can prevent a progressive decline in kidney function and complications.
- Blood pressure control is crucial, and very low targets should be set.
- Cardiovascular risk factors need aggressive management.
- Anemia and bone disease may require treatment before dialysis is necessary.

---

## Key references

Coritsidis GN, Linden E, Stern AS. The role of the primary care physician in managing early stages of chronic kidney disease. *Postgrad Med* 2011;123:177–85.

Flynn C, Bakris GL. Blood pressure targets for patients with diabetes or kidney disease. *Curr Hypertens Rep* 2011;13:452–5.

Levey AS, Bosch JP, Lewis JB et al. Modification of Diet in Renal Disease Study Group. A more accurate method to estimate glomerular filtration rate from serum creatinine: a new prediction equation. *Ann Intern Med* 1999;130:461–70.

Levey AS, Coresh J. Chronic kidney disease. *Lancet* 2012;379:165–80.

Levey AS, Stevens LA, Schmid CH et al. A new equation to estimate glomerular filtration rate. *Ann Intern Med* 2009;150:604–12.

Singh AK. Is there a deleterious effect of erythropoietin in end-stage renal disease? *Kidney Int* 2011;80:569–71.

UK Renal Registry. www.renalreg. com, last accessed 09 May 2013.

www.kidney.org/professionals/kdoqi/ index.cfm, last accessed 09 May 2013.

## Hypertension

Hypertension is the most common chronic disease in the Western world; by the age of 60 years, over 50% of the population will have developed high blood pressure (see *Fast Facts: Hypertension*). Hypertension is even more common among patients with chronic kidney disease (CKD); by the time patients develop end-stage kidney disease (ESKD), over 80% have elevated blood pressure, and hypertension accounts for approximately 20% of all cases of kidney failure. After diabetes mellitus, hypertension is the second leading cause of kidney failure in the USA, though it is less common as a formal cause of ESKD in Europe.

Hypertension is arbitrarily defined as a pressure of 140/90 mmHg or more (Table 5.1); a new category of risk termed prehypertension was created in the USA in guidelines from the Seventh Report of the Joint National Committee on Prevention, Detection, Evaluation and Treatment of High Blood Pressure (JNC 7). After the age of 60 years, most of the population either has hypertension or is at risk of developing it. However, only 59% of these individuals receive treatment, and of these, only 34% are well controlled. The situation is much worse for individuals with CKD; only 14% achieve a blood pressure level of 140/90 mmHg or lower.

TABLE 5.1

**Classification of hypertension**

| Classification | Blood pressure | |
|---|---|---|
| | Systolic (mmHg) | Diastolic (mmHg) |
| Normal | < 120 | < 80 |
| Prehypertension | 120–139 | 80–89 |
| Hypertension | | |
| • stage I | 140–159 | 90–99 |
| • stage II | ≥ 160 | ≥ 100 |

Adapted from the Joint National Committee on the Prevention, Detection, Evaluation and Treatment of High Blood Pressure. *Hypertension* 2003;42:1206–52.

Essential hypertension represents an elevation in systemic arterial blood pressure in the absence of a known etiology and accounts for 90% of cases, with most of the remainder being caused by renal disease. Endocrine or metabolic causes are rare.

Hypertension associated with parenchymal kidney disease represents a potent vicious cycle; it is both a consequence of CKD and a cause of progressive kidney damage. Evidence from many studies shows that treatment of hypertension is crucial to slowing progression of renal disease, particularly among those with significant albuminuria (> 1 g/24 hours).

The major complications associated with elevated blood pressure are an increased risk of cardiovascular and cerebrovascular disease, kidney failure (Figure 5.1), retinopathy and peripheral vascular disease.

Since hypertension is a common chronic condition, the evaluation and treatment of comorbidities associated with hypertension should be an integral part of management. In particular, evidence from the Anglo-Scandinavian Cardiac Outcome Trial (ASCOT) attests to the importance of treating hypertensive patients with a statin. In this study, among hypertensive patients with normal or only moderately raised levels of

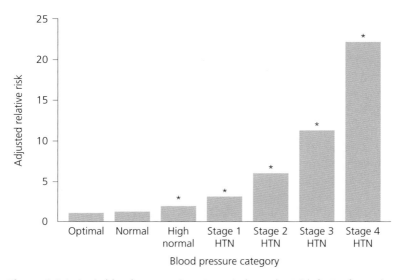

**Figure 5.1** A rise in blood pressure is a strong independent risk factor for end-stage kidney disease. *$p < 0.001$ versus optimal. Data from Klag MJ et al. 1996.

cholesterol, patients receiving atorvastatin were 30% less likely to suffer coronary events and 27% less likely to have a stroke.

**Diagnosis.** The widespread availability of ambulatory electronic and manual devices and the proliferation of automated devices have made the standardization of blood pressure measurement critical to diagnosis and subsequent follow-up. Blood pressure should be measured using the correct size of cuff, with the patient at rest in the correct position, either seated or supine (see *Fast Facts: Hypertension*). Two measurements should be taken at least 2 minutes apart in order to reduce variability. In addition, blood pressure should be measured two or three times, separated by an interval of several weeks before a definitive diagnosis is made, unless the initial measurement is sufficiently high (> 180/100 mmHg) to justify immediate treatment. The UK National Institute for Health and Clinical Excellence (NICE) guidelines indeed suggest that 24-hour ambulatory measurement of blood pressure in primary care is the most clinically and cost-effective method of confirming hypertension by avoiding false positive results and repeat office visits.

**Investigations** should be undertaken to identify the underlying cause, assess the extent of target organ damage, and recognize the presence of comorbid conditions that should influence the aggressiveness of therapy. Routine laboratory evaluation should include urinalysis, blood glucose, complete blood count, urea and electrolytes, lipid profile and an ECG. In most patients, urine protein measurement is a useful indicator of kidney involvement. Screening for microalbuminuria is recommended in type 2 diabetics at the time of diagnosis and in type 1 diabetics at 5 years after the initial diagnosis.

**Management.** Antihypertensive therapy is beneficial in reducing both cardiovascular and renal events, as well as lowering mortality. In patients with CKD, treating hypertension is important in slowing disease progression and in reducing cardiovascular risk. In patients with ESKD, the focus should be directed towards reducing cardiovascular morbidity. Patients with albuminuric CKD (> 500 mg albumin/24 hours) require aggressive management of blood pressure, with a target of less than 130/80 mmHg. A more relaxed target of less than 140/90 mmHg is recommended for patients who are normoalbuminuric.

First-line therapy should comprise lifestyle changes, such as reducing salt intake, moderating alcohol intake, stopping smoking and taking regular exercise, which together can lower blood pressure by 10/5 mmHg. An angiotensin-converting enzyme (ACE) inhibitor or an angiotensin-receptor blocker (ARB) is recommended as first-line therapy in patients with CKD (Figure 5.2). However, usually more than one drug is required, and a β-blocker, a calcium-channel blocker or a diuretic agent can be added. The key features of several commonly used antihypertensive drug classes are shown in Table 5.2. The choice of drugs can be influenced by comorbid conditions, as shown in Table 5.3.

Studies such as the Antihypertensive and Lipid-Lowering Treatment to Prevent Heart Attack Trial (ALLHAT) have shown that achieving optimal blood pressure goals requires multiple drugs, that control of blood pressure using a stepped approach can take up to 2 years and that, in simple essential hypertension, the newer, more expensive drugs do not offer great benefits over thiazide diuretics.

**Renovascular disease** is a remediable form of hypertension and should be excluded in high-risk patients, such as elderly hypertensives with evidence of diffuse atherosclerosis, in refractory or malignant hypertension, in those with 'flash' pulmonary edema and in individuals with an abdominal bruit.

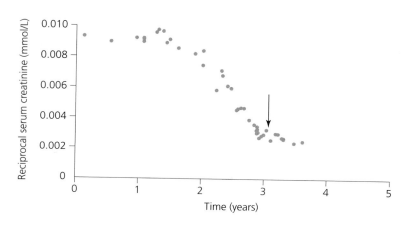

**Figure 5.2** Reciprocal creatinine plot showing how treatment with angiotensin-converting enzyme inhibitor slows the rate of decline in kidney function (arrow).

TABLE 5.2

**Key features of commonly used classes of antihypertensive drugs**

**Angiotensin-converting enzyme inhibitors**
- Renoprotective in chronic kidney disease
- Cardioprotective
- Antiproteinuric
- Generally well tolerated (cough 10–15%, angioedema 0.3%)

**Angiotensin-receptor blockers**
- Renoprotective in chronic kidney disease
- Cardioprotective
- Antiproteinuric
- Generally well tolerated

**β-blockers**
- Lower morbidity and mortality after myocardial infarction
- Potentially diabetogenic
- May mask hypoglycemia
- Lowers high-density lipoprotein cholesterol and raises triglyceride levels

**Calcium-channel blockers**
- Efficacious in multiple settings (blacks, diabetics, elderly)
- Useful in diastolic dysfunction
- Combination with β-blockers can result in severe bradycardia

**Diuretics**
- Preferred agent in congestive heart failure
- Inexpensive
- Associated hypokalemia, lipid abnormalities
- Increased risk of overt diabetes among patients with impaired glucose tolerance (thiazides)

**α-blockers**
- Useful in men with prostatic hypertrophy
- Metabolically neutral

TABLE 5.3

**High-risk comorbid conditions and recommended treatment**

| Comorbid condition | Recommended treatment | | | | |
|---|---|---|---|---|---|
| | Diuretic | β-blocker | ACE inhibitor | ARB | Calcium-channel blocker |
| Heart failure | + | + | + | + | + |
| Post-myocardial infarction | | + | + | + | |
| Coronary artery disease | | + | + | + | |
| Diabetes | | + | + | + | + |
| Chronic kidney disease | | | + | + | + |

ACE, angiotensin-converting enzyme; ARB, angiotensin-receptor blocker.

In young women with hypertension of recent onset, fibromuscular renal artery disease should be excluded. The preferred diagnostic tests include magnetic resonance angiography and ACE-inhibitor renography. Duplex ultrasonography with Doppler flow measurements can be a useful screening test but is rather operator dependent, and in many patients the renal arteries cannot be visualized. The definitive diagnostic tests in almost all patients are still digital subtraction angiography or arteriography (Figure 5.3), but both carry a risk of contrast nephropathy and cholesterol embolization. Magnetic resonance angiography with gadolinium is not recommended in patients with an estimated glomerular filtration rate (GFR) of less than 60 mL/min/1.73m$^2$ because of the risk of gadolinium-associated nephrogenic skin fibrosis, although the risk is very small and possibly dependent on the type of gadolinium used.

Angioplasty (with or without renal artery stenting) does not benefit all patients, as many have diffuse vascular disease including involvement of intrarenal blood vessels, and intervention carries risks (see above). In fact, controlled trials have been unable to demonstrate an overall benefit of intervention compared with aggressive medical therapy. Patients unlikely

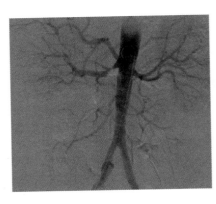

**Figure 5.3** Digital subtraction angiogram showing right renal artery stenosis.

to have a positive response (and perhaps all patients) should receive aggressive medical therapy to control blood pressure, together with statins and acetylsalicylic acid (ASA; aspirin). Surgery to bypass the stenotic lesion is now reserved for lesions that cannot be treated by angioplasty.

**Hypertensive emergencies** are situations in which an immediate reduction in blood pressure is required in order to prevent or treat acute, progressive, target-organ damage. In such cases, a thorough history and physical examination should be undertaken (Table 5.4), including fundoscopy and urine tests for hematuria, proteinuria and red-cell casts. Other investigations should include tests for microangiopathic hemolytic anemia with red-cell fragmentation, kidney dysfunction, evidence of left ventricular hypertrophy and strain, and ischemia on electrocardiography and echocardiography.

The management of a hypertensive emergency requires immediate hospitalization, usually in an intensive care unit, with arterial blood pressure monitoring, central vein catheterization and, occasionally, the use of parenteral drugs such as nitroprusside, glyceryl trinitrate, hydralazine (apresoline), labetalol or fenoldopam (this last not licensed in the UK). Parenteral drugs are rarely needed, since blood pressure can usually be controlled with oral agents such as captopril (fast acting), labetalol (both α- and β-blockade) and clonidine.

**Hypertension during pregnancy** is defined as any rise in systolic blood pressure of more than 30 mmHg or a rise in diastolic blood pressure of more than 15 mmHg above baseline, or the use of antihypertensive agents.

TABLE 5.4

**Clinical features associated with a hypertensive emergency**

- Severe rise in blood pressure (diastolic pressure > 140 mmHg)
- Fundoscopy shows hemorrhages, exudates and papilledema
- Acute kidney injury with albuminuria, hematuria and red-cell casts on urinalysis
- Encephalopathy, headaches, confusion, delirium, visual defects, seizures and coma
- Microangiopathic hemolytic anemia
- Nausea and vomiting

TABLE 5.5

**Classification of hypertension during pregnancy**

| Classification | Definition |
| --- | --- |
| Chronic hypertension | Hypertension present before pregnancy or diagnosed before the 20th week of gestation that persists for > 6 weeks postpartum |
| Pregnancy-induced hypertension | Hypertension detected for the first time after the 20th week of gestation |
| Pre-eclampsia | Hypertension detected for the first time after the 20th week of gestation associated with proteinuria |
| Eclampsia | Pre-eclampsia with seizures that cannot be attributed to other causes |

It is classified according to its presentation (Table 5.5). Chronic hypertension is more common in multiparous women, and is present at the first antenatal visit. On the other hand, pre-eclampsia is more common in primigravidas (in 10% of first pregnancies), and represents an important cause of maternal and perinatal mortality. It usually presents only after 20 weeks of gestation, with or without proteinuria and a raised serum urate. Elevated levels of soluble fms-like tyrosine kinase-1 (sFlt-1 or sVEGFR-1) and endoglin have been reported in pre-eclampsia and have been implicated in disease pathogenesis. Pre-eclampsia may progress to full-blown eclampsia, which is characterized by seizures and also associated with acute kidney injury (AKI). Management of eclampsia comprises immediate delivery, and magnesium sulfate, anticonvulsant and antihypertensive therapy.

Antihypertensive agents must be reviewed in women with renal disease who wish to get pregnant. Methyldopa, labetalol, hydralazine and nifedipine are all safe drugs for treating hypertension in pregnancy, but diuretics should be avoided. ACE inhibitors are contraindicated from the second trimester, but may be important in controlling the progression of CKD. Women may therefore continue to take these as they plan a pregnancy but must stop when pregnant.

## Diabetic nephropathy

Diabetic nephropathy is the most common cause of ESKD in Europe and the USA. Its prevalence is increasing as patients with diabetes are living longer and the complications of diabetes are better controlled. In addition, those who require renal replacement therapy are now accepted onto dialysis programs from which they had previously been excluded. There is considerable racial/ethnic variability in the incidence of diabetes (see *Fast Facts: Diabetes Mellitus*). In the USA, diabetes, and thus ESKD, is more common among native Americans, Hispanics (especially Mexican-Americans), African-Americans, Asian Indians and South Asians (Figure 5.4). ESKD secondary to diabetes mellitus is seen in 45% of patients in the USA, compared with 15% in the UK.

Diabetic nephropathy is defined by the presence of albuminuria. Overt nephropathy is characterized by albuminuria of more than 300 mg/24 hours or 200 µg/minute; in addition, hypertension and kidney dysfunction, with a progressive decline in kidney function over time, may be present. The pathology of nephropathy in type 1 and type 2 diabetes is identical and comprises glomerular hypertrophy, glomerular basement membrane thickening, mesangial matrix accumulation and nodular glomerulosclerosis (Figure 5.5).

**Natural history** (Table 5.6). The earliest clinical evidence of nephropathy is the appearance of microalbuminuria, which is a low but abnormal amount of albumin in the urine (> 30 mg/24 hours or 20 µg/minute). Microalbuminuria can also be detected by an increased albumin:creatinine ratio in a spot urine sample (> 2.5 mg/mmol in men or 3.5 mg/mmol in

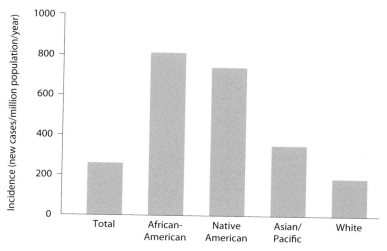

**Figure 5.4** Incidence of end-stage kidney disease (ESKD) in the USA according to racial background (adjusted for age and sex). In the UK, South Asians have a similar excess of ESKD over whites. The excess is mostly due to diabetes.

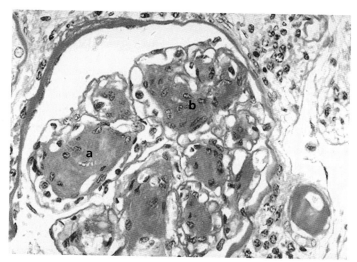

**Figure 5.5** High-power photomicrograph of a glomerulus from a patient with diabetic kidney disease showing (a) mesangial matrix accumulation and (b) Kimmelstiel–Wilson nodules.

67

TABLE 5.6

**Clinical features of diabetic kidney disease by stage**

**Stage 1**

Early, predominantly physiological changes such as hyperfiltration
(GFR supernormal)

**Stage 2**

Progressive thickening of glomerular basement membrane, mesangial
matrix accumulation, glomerular hypertrophy; GFR remains in normal
range and albuminuria is not present

**Stage 3**

Microalbuminuria (30–300 mg/24 hours, urine albumin:creatinine ratio
> 2.5 mg/mmol in men or 3.5 mg/mmol in women) with associated
hypertension

**Stage 4**

Overt nephropathy – urine albumin ≥ 300 mg/24 hours or
albumin:creatinine ratio > 30 mg/mmol, with systolic hypertension,
reduced GFR, continued structural changes, and evidence of glomerular
sclerosis and arteriolar hyalinosis

**Stage 5**

Extensively scarred kidney; patient either in or near end-stage kidney disease

GFR, glomerular filtration rate.

women), which avoids the need for timed urine collections. Patients with
early disease have incipient nephropathy and without specific interventions
may progress to overt or clinical albuminuria over a period of 2–10 years.
Most patients will also develop hypertension, which initially manifests as
the absence of a nocturnal dip in blood pressure, but later becomes
sustained hypertension.

The degree of albuminuria varies quite significantly, but not
uncommonly reaches nephrotic levels (> 3.5 g/24 hours). Once clinical
albuminuria has developed, the GFR often declines relentlessly by
5–15 mL/minute/year. The mortality of patients with diabetic nephropathy
is higher than in other patients because of a four- to eightfold increase in

the rate of cardiovascular complications. In patients with both type 1 and type 2 diabetes, the onset of microalbuminuria is a major risk factor for both cardiovascular disease and mortality, and is also associated with retinopathy, left ventricular cardiac dysfunction and dyslipidemia, as well as hypertension. In all patients with microalbuminuria, other cardiovascular risk factors should be managed by, for example, lowering low-density lipoprotein (LDL) cholesterol, the use of antihypertensive therapy, cessation of smoking and taking exercise.

Diabetic nephropathy in pregnancy can lead to worse hypertension, an increased risk of pre-eclampsia and an accelerated decline in kidney function.

### Screening

*Methods.* Four methods of screening for microalbuminuria are available (Table 5.7). A definitive diagnosis of microalbuminuria requires a positive result from at least two of three samples within a 3–6-month

TABLE 5.7

**Methods of measuring albumin excretion**

| Method | Advantages | Disadvantages |
| --- | --- | --- |
| Urinalysis by microalbumin dipstick | Simple, cheap, rapid | Non-quantitative, small false-negative rate, does not correct for urine concentration |
| Albumin:creatinine ratio in a random spot urine collection | Simple, cheap, quantitative | Morning urine collection preferred because of the known diurnal variation in albumin excretion |
| 24-hour or timed urine collection with measurement of albumin and creatinine | Accurate, inexpensive, quantitative, simultaneous assessment of kidney function by measuring creatinine clearance | Urine collection often incomplete, high non-compliance rate, simultaneous measurement of serum creatinine (for creatinine clearance) |
| Specific immunoassays for urinary albumin | Rapid, simple, portable | Not standardized, expensive |

period, because of high day-to-day variability in urine albumin excretion. Screening dipsticks for microalbumin have acceptable sensitivity (95%) and specificity (93%) when used by trained personnel. All positive tests using reagent strips should be confirmed by more specific methods.

*Type 2 diabetes.* All patients with type 2 diabetes should be screened for incipient or established diabetic nephropathy, because microalbuminuria is present at diagnosis in approximately 25% of patients. If urinalysis is positive for protein (in the absence of infection), it is very likely that the patient has clinical albuminuria (> 300 mg/24 hours), which has important implications in terms of the progression of renal disease and overall cardiovascular risks. Positive urinalysis should be confirmed quantitatively (e.g. spot urine albumin:creatinine ratio), and patients in whom urinalysis is negative for protein require quantitative assessment for microalbuminuria.

*Type 1 diabetes.* In contrast, microalbuminuria is rarely present at the time of diagnosis of type 1 diabetes or before puberty, and therefore screening should begin with the onset of puberty or 5 years after the diagnosis and be performed annually.

**Risk factors.** The major factor influencing the development of diabetic nephropathy is hyperglycemia. Persistent hyperglycemia leads to the development of glycosylated macromolecules and their conversion to advanced glycosylation end products. This process results in thickening of the basement membranes (including the glomerular basement membrane) and accumulation of matrix proteins within the glomeruli.

Although genetic factors predispose individuals to develop diabetes, whether they also influence the rate of progression of the nephropathy remains controversial. The racial and familial distribution of diabetes also suggests a role for as yet undetermined polygenic influences. Other risk factors include male sex and smoking. Apart from glycemic control, the other major factor determining progression through diabetic nephropathy is hypertension (see pages 72–3).

**Prevention and treatment.** Aggressive intervention in patients with either incipient or established nephropathy has been shown unequivocally to prevent progression of renal disease. Strategies include aggressive glycemic control, angiotensin blockade, blood pressure control, protein restriction and smoking cessation (Figure 5.6 and Table 5.8).

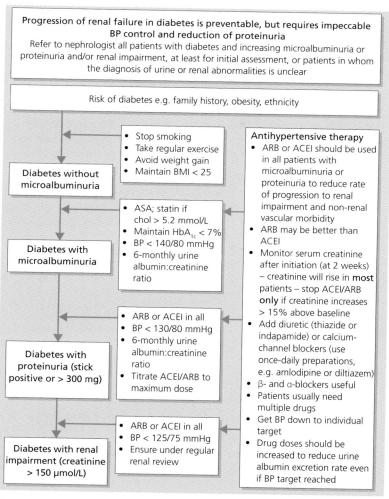

**Figure 5.6** Prevention and treatment of diabetic nephropathy in a community setting. All patients with diabetes and increasing microalbuminuria or proteinuria and/or renal impairment should be referred to a nephrologist, at least for initial assessment, as should patients in whom the diagnosis of urine or kidney abnormalities is unclear. Progression of kidney failure in diabetes is preventable and requires impeccable blood pressure control and reduction of proteinuria. ACEI, angiotensin-converting enzyme inhibitor; ARB, angiotensin-receptor blocker; ASA, acetylsalicylic acid (aspirin); BMI, body mass index; BP, blood pressure; chol, cholesterol.

TABLE 5.8

**Management strategies in diabetic nephropathy**

| Target | Treatment |
|---|---|
| Blood pressure < 130/80 mmHg | ACE inhibitors or ARBs in all patients; most patients need at least two or three drugs, including a diuretic, a calcium antagonist and an α-blocker or β-blocker, with the choice of drug tailored to other comorbidities (e.g. β-blocker in angina, α-blocker in prostatism) |
| Glycosylated hemoglobin < 7% | May need to start insulin; metformin should be discontinued in progressive kidney failure when creatinine > 200 μmol/L |
| Total cholesterol < 5 mmol/L (200 mg/ dL) and low-density lipoprotein cholesterol < 3 mmol/L (130 mg/dL) | All patients with diabetes and renal disease should be managed as if they need secondary prevention for cardiovascular disease and not primary prevention; statins should be started early, and treatment to lower triglycerides may also be required |
| Smoking cessation | Advice and appropriate assistance |
| Obesity | Weight loss and regular exercise |
| Overall cardiovascular risk | Antioxidant vitamins (C and E) may be helpful |
| Diet | Fairly low protein, low saturated fat, low salt, and high fruit and vegetables (if not hyperkalemic) |

ACE, angiotensin-converting enzyme; ARB, angiotensin receptor blocker.

The US Diabetes Control and Complications Trial (DCCT) and the UK Prospective Diabetes Study (UKPDS) have clearly shown that intensive therapy can significantly reduce the risk of the development of microalbuminuria and overt nephropathy in individuals with diabetes. In the UKPDS, there was a 75% reduction in the relative risk of doubling serum creatinine over 12 years.

**Hypertension.** Overwhelming evidence implicates hypertension as a major risk factor in the progression of diabetic nephropathy. Hypertension usually appears during the microalbuminuric phase of disease, although in type 2 diabetes it may result from other causes, such as renovascular disease. Both systolic and diastolic hypertension accelerate the progression of diabetic nephropathy. Aggressive management of hypertension reduces the progression of diabetic renal disease. The VIIth report of the Joint National Committee on the Prevention, Detection, Evaluation and Treatment of High Blood Pressure recommends a target blood pressure in diabetics with renal disease (who are albuminuric) of 130/80 mmHg or lower. Angiotensin blockade should be the first-line therapy, but most patients will require multiple drugs.

The important role of angiotensin blockade in retarding the progression of both type 1 and 2 diabetic nephropathy is now well established. The use of either ACE inhibitors or ARBs should be integrated into the overall antihypertensive management strategy. In addition to reducing systemic blood pressure, angiotensin blockade reduces intraglomerular pressure, thereby protecting the nephron from ongoing damage, and has effects independent of lowering blood pressure. Many studies have shown that in diabetic (and non-diabetic) patients with kidney disease, angiotensin blockade can reduce the level of albuminuria and the rate of progression of renal disease to a greater degree than other antihypertensive agents.

The use of angiotensin blockers may, however, exacerbate hyperkalemia in patients with advanced renal insufficiency and/or hyporeninemic hypoaldosteronism (type IV renal tubular acidosis). Patients with bilateral renal artery stenosis and those with advanced renal disease being treated concurrently with non-steroidal anti-inflammatory drugs (NSAIDs) or who are volume depleted, may experience a rapid decline in kidney function when started on an ACE inhibitor; it is likely that ARBs have a similar effect. This is usually reversible when the drug is discontinued.

As a high proportion of patients progress from microalbuminuria to overt nephropathy and subsequently to ESKD, ACE inhibitors or ARBs are recommended for all patients with microalbuminuria. The effect of an ACE inhibitor appears to be a class effect, so the choice of agent may depend on cost and compliance issues; the same is probably true for ARBs.

*Protein restriction* has been shown to be effective in retarding progression of renal disease in several animal models by reducing glomerular hyperfiltration and intraglomerular pressures. While small studies in humans with diabetic nephropathy have shown that protein restriction (0.6 g/kg/day) confers a moderate benefit in retarding progression, restricting protein in diabetics is hard to achieve and may lead to protein malnutrition. Nevertheless, the general consensus is to prescribe a protein intake of approximately the adult recommended dietary allowance of 0.8 g/kg/day (10% of daily calories) in patients with overt nephropathy.

## Key points – hypertension and diabetic nephropathy

- Hypertension is both an important cause and a consequence of renal disease.
- Blood pressure targets are less than 130/80 mmHg or lower in the presence of albuminuria (> 500 mg/day) and less than 140/90 mmHg in the absence of albuminuria.
- Pregnant women with significant renal impairment are likely to have hypertension, pre-eclampsia and premature labor.
- For optimal renal protection in patients with chronic kidney disease, angiotensin blockade with an ACE inhibitor or an ARB is recommended.
- Medications, particularly antihypertensive agents, require careful review in pregnant women with renal disease.
- The earliest clinical evidence of nephropathy is microalbuminuria, which can be tested by an increased albumin:creatinine ratio in a spot urine sample (> 2.5 mg/mol in men or 3.5 mg/mol in women).
- All patients with type 2 diabetes should be screened for incipient or established diabetic nephropathy, as microalbuminuria is present in about 25% of patients at diagnosis.
- Microalbuminuria is rarely present at diagnosis in type 1 diabetes; these patients should therefore be screened at the onset of puberty or 5 years after diagnosis, then annually.
- The major risk factor for development of diabetic nephropathy is hyperglycemia.
- Aggressive intervention in patients with incipient or established nephropathy unequivocally prevents progression of renal disease.
- Treatment strategies for diabetic nephropathy include aggressive glycemic control, angiotensin blockade, blood pressure control, protein restriction and smoking cessation.

## Key references

Aronow WS, Fleg JL, Pepine CJ et al ACCF/AHA 2011 expert consensus document on hypertension in the elderly: a report of the American College of Cardiology Foundation Task Force on Clinical Expert Consensus Documents developed in collaboration with the American Academy of Neurology, American Geriatrics Society, American Society for Preventive Cardiology, American Society of Hypertension, American Society of Nephrology, Association of Black Cardiologists, and European Society of Hypertension. *J Am Soc Hypertens* 2011;5:259–352.

Bakris GL. Recognition, pathogenesis, and treatment of different stages of nephropathy in patients with type 2 diabetes mellitus. *Mayo Clin Proc* 2011; 86:444–56.

Flynn C, Bakris GL. Blood pressure targets for patients with diabetes or kidney disease. *Curr Hypertens Rep* 2011;13:452–5.

Higgins JR, de Swiet M. Blood-pressure measurement and classification in pregnancy. *Lancet* 2001;357:131–5.

JNC7. *The Seventh Report of the Joint National Committee on Prevention, Detection, Evaluation, and Treatment of High Blood Pressure*, 2004. Available at www. nhlbi.nih.gov/guidelines/ hypertension/jnc7full.htm, last accessed 09 May 2013.

Jun M, Perkovic V, Cass A. Intensive glycemic control and renal outcome. *Contrib Nephrol* 2011;170:196–208.

Khouri Y, Steigerwalt SP, Alsamara M, McCullough PA. What is the ideal blood pressure goal for patients with stage III or higher chronic kidney disease? *Curr Cardiol Rep* 2011;13:492–501.

Klag MJ, Whelton PK, Randall BL et al. Blood pressure and end-stage renal disease in men. *N Engl J Med* 1996;334:13–18.

MacGregor GA, Kaplan NM. *Fast Facts: Hypertension*, 4th edn. Oxford: Health Press, 2010.

Reutens AT, Atkins RC. Epidemiology of diabetic nephropathy. *Contrib Nephrol* 2011;170:1–7.

Ritz E. Limitations and future treatment options in type 2 diabetes with renal impairment. *Diabetes Care* 2011;34 Suppl 2:S330–4.

Scobie IN, Samaras K. *Fast Facts: Diabetes Mellitus*, 4th edn. Oxford: Health Press, 2012.

www.kidney.org/professionals/ kdoqi/index.cfm, last accessed 09 May 2013.

Glomerulonephritis is the term used to describe abnormalities of the glomerulus resulting from a variety of immune and inflammatory mechanisms. Glomerulonephritis is often described as primary, when there is no associated disease elsewhere, or secondary, when glomerular involvement is part of a systemic disease. This chapter considers primary glomerulonephritis; secondary glomerulonephritis is discussed in the context of systemic disease in Chapter 7.

Primary glomerulonephritis may be described or classified according to the clinical syndrome produced (e.g. nephrotic syndrome), the histopathological appearance (e.g. membranous nephropathy) or the underlying etiology (relevant mainly in secondary causes). Unfortunately, there is no direct correlation between the clinical syndrome produced and the pathological description. In most glomerular diseases, the natural history and response to treatment have been defined with respect to the histopathological diagnosis (except for nephrotic syndrome in children), so a pathological description is preferred when considering management.

## Presentation

Glomerulonephritis presents in a limited number of ways, depending on the nature and severity of the glomerular injury.

- Mild disease can present with asymptomatic hematuria and/or proteinuria. If proteinuria becomes heavy, leading to hypoalbuminemia and fluid retention, it is described as the nephrotic syndrome.
- More severe, acute forms of glomerulonephritis may present with 'acute nephritic syndrome', which involves hematuria (sometimes macroscopic), albuminuria, a fall in glomerular filtration rate (GFR), salt and water retention, and hypertension.
- Rapidly progressive glomerulonephritis describes a rapid loss of kidney function, such that the patient will be in end-stage kidney disease (ESKD) within weeks or months.
- Chronic glomerulonephritis involves a much slower deterioration in kidney function, usually over several years, accompanied by hematuria, albuminuria and hypertension.

Hypertension may also be the presenting feature of some forms of glomerulonephritis.

## Pathological classification

Except in the mildest cases, or in nephrotic syndrome in children, the suspicion of glomerulonephritis should lead to kidney biopsy. The commonly used pathological classification depends on light microscopy, but immunohistochemistry and electron microscopy provide additional information and may give clues as to the etiology. A single glomerulus is depicted in Figure 6.1.

### Histological patterns

*Minimal change disease.* Light microscopy is virtually normal, but there is widespread effacement of the epithelial cell foot processes on the outside of the glomerular basement membrane. Immunofluorescence is generally negative.

*Focal segmental glomerulosclerosis.* Some of the glomeruli show segmental scarring, together with foot process effacement as in minimal change disease.

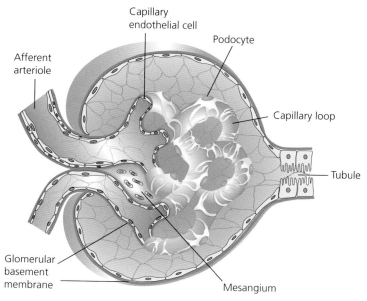

**Figure 6.1** Structure of a single glomerulus.

*Membranous nephropathy* is characterized by widespread thickening of the glomerular basement membrane. Immunofluorescence reveals granular deposits of immunoglobulin (Ig) and complement.

*Mesangiocapillary glomerulonephritis (MCGN)* is also known as membranoproliferative glomerulonephritis. There is proliferation of mesangial cells, an increase in mesangial matrix and thickening of the glomerular basement membrane. MCGN can be subdivided according to the appearance on electron microscopy. Type 1 has electron dense subendothelial deposits of immunoglobulin and complement, while type 2 has characteristic linear 'dense deposits' along the glomerular basement membrane.

*Mesangial proliferative nephritis.* Mesangial cell proliferation combined with matrix expansion occurs. It is most often seen in the context of IgA deposition, when it is known as IgA nephropathy. Other immunoglobulins and complement components may also be present.

*Diffuse proliferative glomerulonephritis* is characterized by widespread hypercellularity, caused by both infiltrating inflammatory cells and proliferation of endothelial and mesangial cells. There is generally deposition of immunoglobulins and complement around the capillary loops.

*Focal and segmental proliferative glomerulonephritis* is generally secondary to systemic disease (see Chapter 7). There is often associated segmental necrosis of the capillary loops, which is followed by crescent formation. The term crescentic glomerulonephritis is used when there is an accumulation of cells outside the capillary loops, but within Bowman's capsule.

*Crescentic glomerulonephritis* (Figure 6.2) may occur as part of the evolution of certain forms of primary glomerulonephritis (e.g. IgA nephropathy or MCGN), but is more often seen in conditions such as Goodpasture's syndrome and systemic vasculitis. A condition previously described as idiopathic crescentic glomerulonephritis is now recognized as generally being due to renal limited vasculitis. The immunofluorescence findings are most informative in the diagnosis of crescentic glomerulonephritis (Table 6.1).

**Investigations** consist of an assessment of the severity of glomerular injury, together with a search for the cause (Table 6.2).

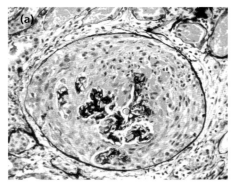

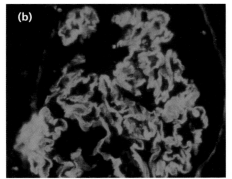

**Figure 6.2** (a) Histological section of a kidney biopsy showing a single glomerulus from a patient with rapidly progressive glomerulonephritis and antineutrophil cytoplasm antibody-associated crescentic nephritis (the glomerulus is completely compressed by a crescent of cells). (b) Immunohistology of kidney biopsy showing antibody deposition on glomerular capillaries in anti-glomerular basement membrane disease (Goodpasture's syndrome).

TABLE 6.1

**Classification of rapidly progressive glomerulonephritis based on immunofluorescence findings on kidney biopsy**

| Immunofluorescence finding | Disorder |
| --- | --- |
| Linear deposits | Anti-glomerular basement membrane disease |
| Granular deposits | Primary or secondary immune complex glomerulonephritis |
| No (or few) deposits | Antineutrophil cytoplasm antibody-associated glomerulonephritis |

## Clinical features and management

It is possible to provide only a brief outline here; further information should be sought from expert sources in order to manage patients.

TABLE 6.2

**Investigation of glomerulonephritis**

| Investigation | Comment |
|---|---|
| Urine dipstick and microscopy | In glomerulonephritis, hematuria and/or albuminuria will be found and, in some forms, red-cell casts |
| Urine albumin quantification | Measured in 24-hour urine sample or by albumin:creatinine ratio |
| Glomerular filtration rate | Determined from serum creatinine and patient characteristics using a formula, or by 24-hour creatinine clearance |
| Biochemistry | Serum albumin low in nephrotic syndrome; high potassium, low bicarbonate and high phosphate in kidney failure |
| Glucose | To exclude diabetes |
| Serum immunoglobulins, serum and urine protein electrophoresis, serum free light chains | To exclude myeloma |
| Serum complement | Low in systemic lupus erythematosus and cryoglobulinemia and some forms of primary glomerulonephritis |
| Antineutrophil cytoplasm antibody, anti-glomerular basement membrane antibodies and antinuclear antibodies | Found in the associated disease |

**Minimal change disease** accounts for most cases of nephrotic syndrome in children, and about 20% of cases in adults. It is associated with atopy in children and may be related to underlying Hodgkin's disease in adults. It usually responds to a course of high-dose prednisolone, but relapse is frequent. Relapsing disease may go into remission following treatment with prednisolone and cyclophosphamide. Alternatively, ciclosporin or tacrolimus can be used, but relapses may occur when the drug is discontinued. Although severe nephrotic syndrome has its own complications (e.g. thrombotic episodes, infection), minimal change disease does not progress to ESKD.

**Focal segmental glomerulosclerosis** is a common cause of nephrotic syndrome in older children and younger adults; it may be associated with hematuria. About 50% of patients may respond to a course of high-dose prednisolone, although treatment for up to 4 months is often required in adults. If this is unsuccessful, some patients may respond to the addition of cyclophosphamide or rituximab; ciclosporin or tacrolimus can also be used to reduce albuminuria. Focal segmental glomerulosclerosis often progresses to ESKD over several years, but progression may be curtailed by treatment with corticosteroids.

A variant known as 'collapsing glomerulopathy' is associated with infection with human immunodeficiency virus (HIV). Antiretroviral therapy may be effective, and some patients respond to additional corticosteroids.

**Membranous nephropathy** is the most common cause of nephrotic syndrome in older adults. Hematuria is rare. Although many cases are idiopathic, it may also be secondary to systemic lupus erythematosus (SLE), hepatitis B, malignancy, or the use of gold or penicillamine. Antibodies to the phospholipase A2 receptor ($PLA_2R$) are often detected in idiopathic membranous nephropathy, and may be pathogenic. The idiopathic form may respond to a treatment regimen involving alternate months of corticosteroids and chlorambucil or cyclophosphamide (often known as the 'Ponticelli regimen'), or to ciclosporin or tacrolimus. There are recent reports of responses to rituximab. Membranous nephropathy progresses to ESKD in 30–50% of patients.

**Mesangiocapillary glomerulonephritis** is an uncommon disorder that can present as nephrotic syndrome or nephritic syndrome in children and young adults. Secondary forms of the disease are associated with hepatitis C with or without cryoglobulins, other chronic infections and SLE. Some cases are related to genetic or acquired dysregulation of complement, and these are being described as C3 nephropathy. Despite the lack of evidence from controlled studies, nephrotic patients with primary MCGN are often treated with corticosteroids.

**Immunoglobulin A nephropathy** is the most common form of glomerulonephritis worldwide. It often presents with macroscopic hematuria, which may be precipitated within a few days by an upper respiratory tract infection. It is also detected as asymptomatic hematuria and/or albuminuria, and can present with nephrotic syndrome. Some studies suggest that a course of high-dose prednisolone can reduce albuminuria and delay renal impairment. In patients with deteriorating kidney function, the addition of immunosuppressive drugs has been proposed. There are conflicting reports of the benefit of high-dose fish oil, but one US study suggests slowing of renal impairment. Although progression is slow, 20–30% of patients may eventually develop ESKD. The renal lesion of Henoch–Schönlein purpura is similar to that of IgA nephropathy, and this may be a variant of the same disease.

**Diffuse proliferative glomerulonephritis** generally presents with an acute nephritic syndrome 2 or more weeks after an infection. Classically, the disease is caused by streptococcal infection, either of the pharynx or the skin. Although rare in developed countries, poststreptococcal glomerulonephritis remains common in the developing world. Many other bacterial and viral causes have now been described. Almost all children will recover without treatment (other than antibiotics for the infection), but a small proportion of adults may develop chronic kidney disease (CKD).

**Crescentic glomerulonephritis** should be treated according to the underlying cause. So-called idiopathic crescentic glomerulonephritis is now widely regarded as a form of antineutrophil cytoplasm antibody (ANCA)-positive vasculitis limited to the kidney. It presents with the clinical syndrome of rapidly progressive glomerulonephritis. Without treatment, the disease progresses to ESKD within a few weeks or months, but prednisolone and cyclophosphamide are generally effective in patients before severe kidney damage occurs. The addition of plasma exchange or pulse doses of methylprednisolone is recommended in patients with advanced renal disease. Indeed, evidence suggests that plasma exchange may be the more effective approach.

**Goodpasture's syndrome** is due to autoantibodies directed against the $\alpha3$ chain of type IV collagen, which is a major structural component of the glomerular basement membrane. This collagen is also found in the alveolar basement membrane and accounts for the pulmonary hemorrhage that is seen in 50% of patients with this disorder (Figure 6.3).

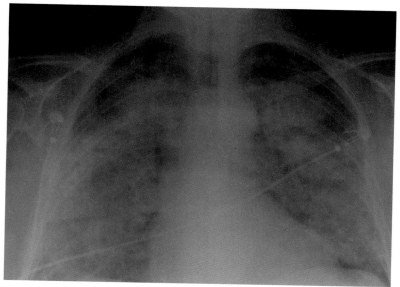

**Figure 6.3** Chest radiograph showing extensive pulmonary hemorrhage in a patient with Goodpasture's syndrome.

The syndrome presents with rapidly progressive glomerulonephritis, usually leading to kidney failure within 6 months if untreated. Treatment with prednisolone and cyclophosphamide, combined with plasma exchange to remove circulating anti-glomerular basement membrane antibodies rapidly, is generally effective if started before renal disease is advanced. However, patients will seldom recover kidney function once they start dialysis. It is extremely rare for patients to relapse, and the long-term outcome is good following successful treatment.

## Key points – glomerulonephritis

- Glomerulonephritis should be considered in all patients with urine abnormalities.
- Urgent investigations are needed to determine the precise type.
- Treatments are available for most categories of glomerulonephritis.
- Crescentic glomerulonephritis requires urgent and aggressive immunosuppression.

## Key references

Beck LH Jr, Bonegio RG, Lambeau G et al. M-type phospholipase A2 receptor as target antigen in idiopathic membranous nephropathy. *N Engl J Med* 2009;361:11–21.

Beck LH Jr, Salant DJ. Glomerular and tubulointerstitial diseases. *Prim Care* 2008;35:265–96, vi.

D'Agati VD, Kaskel FJ, Falk RJ. Focal segmental glomerulosclerosis. *N Engl J Med* 2011;365:2398–411.

Jennette JC, Falk RJ. Glomerular clinicopathologic syndromes. In: Greenberg A (ed). *NKF Primer on Kidney Diseases*, 5th edn. Philadelphia: Saunders Elsevier, 2009:148–69.

Salama AD, Pusey CD. Goodpasture's syndrome and other anti-GBM disease. In: Greenberg A (ed). *NKF Primer on Kidney Diseases*, 5th edn. Philadelphia: Saunders Elsevier, 2009:186–90.

Suzuki H, Kiryluk K, Novak J et al. The pathophysiology of IgA nephropathy. *J Am Soc Nephrol* 2011;22:1795–803.

Tarzi RM, Cook HT, Pusey CD. Crescentic glomerulonephritis: new aspects of pathogenesis. *Semin Nephrol* 2011;31:361–8.

Glomerular or tubular involvement may be a major feature of systemic autoimmune diseases, and may result from the deposition of abnormal proteins in dysproteinemias. Diabetic nephropathy is becoming the commonest cause of kidney failure in developed countries; this is discussed in Chapter 5.

## Systemic lupus erythematosus

Systemic lupus erythematosus (SLE) is a multisystem autoimmune disease that is most common in young women and often affects the joints, skin, nervous system and kidneys. Approximately 50% of patients with SLE will eventually develop kidney disease. This may affect the glomeruli directly, small blood vessels within the kidney or the interstitium. A variety of forms of lupus nephritis can be identified by standard light microscopy.

- class I – minimal mesangial lupus nephritis
- class II – mesangial proliferative lupus nephritis
- class III – focal lupus nephritis
- class IV-S – diffuse segmental lupus nephritis
- class IV-G – global lupus nephritis
- class V – membranous lupus nephritis
- class VI – advanced sclerosing lupus nephritis.

In classes I and II, mesangial deposits of immunoglobulin (Ig) with or without complement are found. In classes III and IV, there is widespread deposition of various classes of Ig and complement along the capillary walls. In class V, subepithelial deposits predominate, as in primary membranous nephropathy. Stage VI, the final stage, represents advanced sclerosing lupus nephritis, with more than 90% sclerosis of the glomeruli.

**Clinical features.** Lupus nephritis can present with any of the clinical syndromes described earlier, depending on the severity of glomerular injury. Serology will often show elevated levels of anti-DNA antibodies and anti-C1q antibodies, together with reduced levels of serum complement C4 and/or C3. The erythrocyte sedimentation rate (ESR) is often raised, but the C-reactive protein may be normal unless an accompanying infection is present.

In pregnancy, SLE confers a a high risk of spontaneous abortion and problems for the fetus (e.g. neonatal lupus, heart block).

**Treatment** depends on the severity of the kidney lesion. There is good evidence for using a combination of prednisolone and pulsed cyclophosphamide as initial therapy, followed by azathioprine for maintenance in class III and IV lupus nephritis. Several studies suggest that mycophenolate mofetil together with prednisolone is at least as effective as, and less toxic than, cyclophosphamide. Rituximab is also emerging as a potentially useful therapy, but is not yet supported by clinical trial data. Consequently, in most centers combination therapy with prednisolone and mycophenolate mofetil is now preferred first-line therapy to induce remission. Since the disease runs a relapsing and remitting course, maintenance therapy, often with low-dose prednisolone and mycophenolate mofetil, is generally required. Azathioprine is safe in pregnancy and can be an effective alternative.

## Primary systemic vasculitis

Primary vasculitides cause necrotizing inflammation of the blood vessels, and can be classified according to the size of blood vessel they affect (Figure 7.1).

Primary vasculitides affecting small blood vessels, which include granulomatosis with polyangiitis (Wegener's) (GPA), microscopic polyangiitis and, less commonly, Churg–Strauss syndrome, often cause glomerulonephritis. In some patients, vasculitis appears to be restricted to the kidney. These disorders show a slight male predominance and are more common in the elderly. The characteristic glomerular lesion is a focal and segmental necrotizing glomerulonephritis, which often progresses to crescent formation. There are no or scanty immune deposits.

**Clinical features.** Patients generally present with a rapidly progressive glomerulonephritis, although in some patients there may be repeated episodes of less severe renal disease, leading to glomerular scarring together with active lesions. Antineutrophil cytoplasm antibodies (ANCAs) have a high sensitivity and specificity in the diagnosis of these diseases, and can be divided according to the pattern seen on human neutrophils by immunofluorescence (Figure 7.2). Perinuclear ANCAs (P-ANCAs; Figure 7.2a) are often associated with reactivity against myeloperoxidase, and are more commonly seen in microscopic polyangiitis and renal-limited vasculitis. Cytoplasmic ANCAs (C-ANCAs; Figure 7.2b) are usually the result of reactivity against proteinase 3, and are most often associated with GPA.

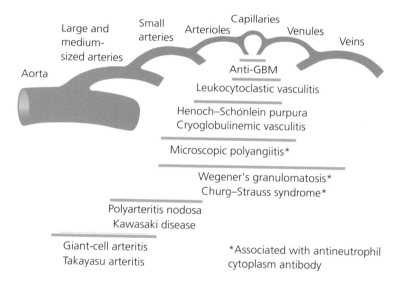

Figure 7.1 Classification of systemic vasculitis. GBM, glomerular basement membrane.

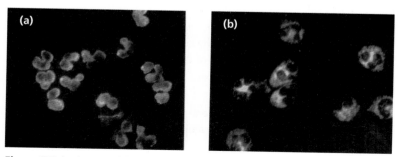

Figure 7.2 Antineutrophil cytoplasm antibody (ANCA) as shown by immuno-fluorescence using neutrophils: (a) perinuclear ANCA; (b) cytoplasmic ANCA.

**Treatment.** Most patients respond well to treatment with prednisolone and cyclophosphamide. Recent studies suggest that rituximab is as effective as cyclophosphamide for induction therapy. Once remission has been induced (generally within 3 months), cyclophosphamide may be replaced by azathioprine for maintenance therapy. Mycophenolate mofetil can be used in those intolerant of azathioprine. Patients with severe kidney failure or other life-threatening features of disease are generally treated with additional intravenous methylprednisolone and/or plasma exchange. There is evidence that plasma exchange may be more effective than methylprednisolone in salvaging kidney function in patients with advanced kidney failure. With aggressive treatment, most patients, even those on dialysis, will recover kidney function.

## Hemolytic uremic syndrome

Hemolytic uremic syndrome (HUS) is a form of thrombotic microangiopathy, with a tendency to affect the kidney. Kidney histology reveals widespread intraglomerular thrombi, together with an occlusive vasculopathy. Kidney involvement is often accompanied by hematologic and neurological manifestations. There is some clinical overlap with thrombotic thrombocytopenic purpura (TTP), though different disease mechanisms are involved.

**Children.** HUS in children is commonly related to gastrointestinal infection with *Escherichia coli* O157, which produces a verotoxin thought to damage endothelial cells. Most affected children will recover spontaneously, though some are left with renal impairment. The role of specific treatment in this so-called D+ HUS is unclear.

**Adults** may develop HUS sporadically (without obvious infection), on a familial basis or related to a variety of drugs. Some adults with HUS have been shown to have deficiencies in complement regulatory proteins, such as factor H. The principle of treatment is to replace deficient plasma components, together with the removal of potentially harmful abnormal components. This is achieved by plasma exchange with fresh frozen plasma, often accompanied by corticosteroids to reduce inflammation. The use of eculizumab, a monoclonal antibody to complement protein C5, is also being investigated. No good trials of treatment have been reported in HUS, though plasma exchange with fresh frozen plasma has been shown to be effective in TTP.

## Systemic sclerosis

Systemic sclerosis may affect the kidney by causing an obstructive vasculopathy of small renal arteries – so-called 'scleroderma kidney'.

**Clinical features.** Systemic sclerosis of the kidney presents with subacute or acute renal impairment. Kidney failure may be compounded by vasospasm in addition to the structural lesions. Although systemic features of scleroderma are generally present (e.g. thickening of the skin, telangiectasia, esophageal dysfunction), kidney involvement may occasionally be the presenting feature.

**Treatment** with angiotensin-converting enzyme (ACE) inhibitors improves the renal outcome. Prostacyclin may relieve spasm of intrarenal arteries.

## Sarcoidosis

Sarcoidosis is a disease of unknown etiology, characterized by granulomatous inflammation of a number of organs, including the lungs and kidneys. The typical kidney lesion is a granulomatous tubulointerstitial nephritis, which can lead to functional impairment. This will generally respond to treatment with corticosteroids. Sarcoidosis may also lead to hypercalcemia, which can itself cause kidney dysfunction.

## Cryoglobulinemia

Cryoglobulins are immunoglobulins that precipitate in the cold; three major types have been described (Table 7.1). Type I cryoglobulins are more likely to result in kidney damage through high viscosity or intravascular deposition. Treatment of acute kidney injury (AKI) in type I cryoglobulinemia generally involves plasma exchange to reduce paraprotein levels, together with appropriate chemotherapy.

Type II cryoglobulins often lead to mesangiocapillary glomerulonephritis (MCGN). Clinical features commonly include a purpuric rash, arthralgia and peripheral neuropathy. Many cases are

TABLE 7.1

**Classification of cryoglobulinemia**

| Cryoglobulin | | Associated disease |
|---|---|---|
| Type I | Monoclonal, usually IgM, occasionally IgG, rarely IgA | Lymphoproliferative diseases (e.g. myeloma, Waldenström's macroglobulinemia, non-Hodgkin's lymphoma) |
| Type II | Mixture of monoclonal rheumatoid factor (usually IgM) and polyclonal Ig | Lymphoproliferative diseases; hepatitis C or rarely other chronic infections |
| Type III | Mixture of polyclonal rheumatoid factor and polyclonal Ig | Malignancy, chronic infections, autoimmune disease (e.g. systemic lupus erythematosus), chronic liver disease |

Ig, immunoglobulin.

associated with hepatitis C infection, when treatment with appropriate antiviral drugs is recommended. Plasma exchange may be helpful in removing circulating cryoglobulins in the most severe disease, and can be combined with prednisolone and cyclophosphamide therapy. Rituximab is also reported to be effective. Type III cryoglobulins are generally related to an underlying autoimmune disease or chronic infection. They rarely cause severe renal disease. Treatment involves management of the underlying disorder.

## Myeloma and monoclonal dysproteinemias

Multiple myeloma may affect the kidney in many different ways (Table 7.2). Cast nephropathy appears to be an increasingly common cause of AKI or subacute kidney failure, particularly in the elderly. Adequate hydration and correction of hypercalcemia and other metabolic abnormalities are crucial. There is some evidence that plasma exchange (to reduce paraprotein levels) is beneficial, accompanied by chemotherapy to treat the myeloma.

TABLE 7.2

**Causes of kidney dysfunction in myeloma**

- Light chain cast nephropathy
- Light and heavy chain deposition disease
- AL (light chain) amyloidosis
- Cryoglobulinemia
- Hypercalcemic nephropathy
- Acute urate nephropathy
- Acute interstitial nephritis
- Pyelonephritis
- Obstructive uropathy

## Amyloidosis

The term amyloid is used to describe insoluble deposits of protein formed by the association of amyloid P component, together with other proteins that possess characteristic physicochemical properties. The commonest forms affecting the kidney are AL amyloid, in which Ig light chains are involved, and AA amyloid, in which amyloid A protein produced by chronic inflammation is involved. More rarely, mutations in other serum proteins can lead to amyloidosis of a familial nature (e.g. mutations in transthyretin, lysosyme, apolipoprotein E).

Amyloid deposition in the kidney commonly results in nephrotic syndrome, usually associated with progressive renal impairment. Deposition in other organs depends on the type of amyloid, but there is commonly damage to the liver, spleen, heart and nervous system. Reducing the load of amyloid precursor proteins may allow resolution of the condition (slowly). This might be achieved by appropriate chemotherapy for dysproteinemia in AL amyloid, or by tight control of the underlying inflammatory disease in AA amyloid.

## Atherosclerotic renovascular disease

Atherosclerotic renovascular disease is an increasingly important cause of established kidney failure in the elderly. Atheroma of the renal arteries is commonly seen as an extension of aortic disease, so atheromatous renal artery stenosis is usually proximal (Figure 7.3).

The natural history is generally of progression. Atherosclerosis may lead to kidney dysfunction by occlusion of the arterial lumen, though this requires a greater than 70% stenosis. Perhaps of greater importance, atheroma of the renal artery can lead to cholesterol embolization of intrarenal vessels or glomeruli, which often causes irreversible kidney failure.

Radiological intervention using angioplasty, with or without stenting, is generally successful in relieving renal artery stenosis. Current indications for radiological intervention are summarized in Table 7.3. The long-term effects on kidney function have not been adequately studied, although recent trials have failed to show major benefit on outcomes including renal function, the need for dialysis or blood pressure control.

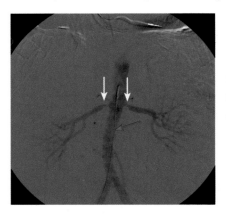

**Figure 7.3** Bilateral renal artery stenosis (white arrows) and atheromatous aorta (red arrow).

TABLE 7.3

**Indications for radiological intervention in atherosclerotic renovascular disease**

Significant stenosis (> 60%) with:

- Resistant hypertension
- Flash pulmonary edema
- Renal impairment related to angiotensin-converting enzyme inhibitors
- Progressively declining kidney function
- Single functioning kidney

## Key points – systemic disease

- Systemic lupus erythematosus (SLE) commonly causes kidney disease, which can be severe and requires immunosuppression.
- Vasculitis is common in the elderly and can be successfully treated if diagnosed early.
- Long-term treatment is usually needed for both vasculitis and SLE with kidney involvement.
- Atheromatous renal vascular disease is very common and reflects widespread arterial pathology.

## Key references

Berden AE, Ferrario F, Hagen EC et al. Histopathologic classification of ANCA-associated glomerulonephritis. *J Am Soc Nephrol* 2010;21:1628–36.

Chen M, Kallenberg CG. ANCA-associated vasculitides – advances in pathogenesis and treatment. *Nat Rev Rheumatol* 2010;6:653–64.

Houssiau FA. Toward better treatment for lupus nephritis. *N Engl J Med* 2011;365:1929–30.

Jeannette JC, Falk RJ, Bacon PA et al. 2012 revised International Chapel Hill Consensus Conference Nomenclature of Vaculitides. *Arthritis Rheum* 2013;65:1–11.

Jeannette JC, Falk RJ, Gasim AH et al. Pathogenesis of antineutrophil cytoplasmic autoantibody vasculitis. *Curr Opin Nephrol Hypertens* 2011;20:263–70.

Merlini G, Seldin DC, Gertz MA. Amyloidosis: pathogenesis and new therapeutic options. *J Clin Oncol* 2011;29:1924–33.

Rutgers A, Sanders JS, Stegeman CA, Kallenberg CG. Pauci-immune necrotizing glomerulonephritis. *Rheum Dis Clin North Am* 2010;36:559–72.

Textor SC. Ischemic nephropathy: where are we now? *J Am Soc Nephrol* 2004;15:1974–82.

Walters G, Willis NS, Craig JC. Interventions for renal vasculitis in adults. *Cochrane Database Syst Rev* 2008;CD003232.

Weening JJ, D'Agati VD, Schwartz MM et al. The classification of glomerulonephritis in systemic lupus erythematosus revisited. *Kidney Int* 2004;65:521–30.

## Autosomal-dominant polycystic kidney disease

Autosomal-dominant polycystic kidney disease (APKD) is a common inherited multisystem disease in which patients develop multiple bilateral kidney cysts, cysts in other organs and non-cystic renal manifestations (Figure 8.1).

**Pathophysiology.** Most patients (85–90%) have a mutation in the *PKD1* gene, which encodes the protein polycystin. Mutations in a second gene, *PKD2*, can also cause APKD. The precise function of the proteins encoded by *PKD1* and *PKD2* has not been clarified, though they are likely to play a role in cell–cell and cell–matrix interactions, and possibly as a transmembrane ion channel. Cysts arise from focal dilatation of the tubules.

**Clinical features of APKD** are summarized in Table 8.1. APKD affects about 1 in 1000 people, making it one of the commonest inherited diseases. It is a common cause of end-stage kidney disease (ESKD); however, progression is slow in most patients, and not inevitable.

**Diagnosis.** Cysts are easily identified by ultrasound examination. Cysts are not commonly seen in the fetus or in children. They are, however, found in a number of conditions other than APKD, such as simple cysts, tuberous sclerosis and von Hippel–Lindau disease. The absence of cysts in young people does not exclude the diagnosis, because they can form late in life, and screening of asymptomatic individuals is therefore not recommended before the age of 20 years. If negative, a scan should then be repeated at

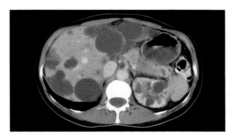

**Figure 8.1** CT scan showing polycystic kidneys and liver in autosomal-dominant polycystic kidney disease.

TABLE 8.1

**Clinical features of autosomal-dominant polycystic kidney disease**

| Feature | Comment |
|---------|---------|
| Kidney cyst formation | • Causes pain, mass effects, gastrointestinal disturbance, cyst hemorrhage and hematuria |
| Urinary tract infection | • Presents as cystitis, pyelonephritis, cyst infection or perinephric abscess<br>• Usually caused by Gram-negative organisms<br>• Mainly affects women |
| Kidney stones | • Occur in 20% of patients<br>• Usually uric acid or calcium oxalate |
| Hypertension | • Found in 75% of patients before onset of kidney failure<br>• Associated with kidney size<br>• Significantly increases the risk of kidney failure |
| Kidney failure | • 50% of patients develop end-stage kidney disease by the age of 50–70 years<br>• Earlier onset in those with *PKD1* mutations |
| Polycystic liver | • Occurs in 25–70% of patients (increasing with age)<br>• More common in women<br>• Causes symptoms from massive enlargement of liver or mass effect |
| Intracranial aneurysm | • Occurs in 8% of patients, and family history common<br>• Screening not generally advised because aneurysms are small, unlikely to rupture and require no treatment |
| Mitral valve prolapse | • Common, but rarely significant |

5-yearly intervals in individuals with a family history. Genetic diagnosis by mutation analysis or linkage analysis is possible, but not always available, and may require blood samples from family members.

**Treatment.** No specific treatments are available. Pain may require strong analgesics, and nephrotoxic agents should be avoided. Cyst hemorrhage is usually self limiting. Upper tract infection should be treated with antibiotics that will penetrate cysts (fluoroquinolones). Stones are managed as in patients without APKD (see Chapter 10). Hypertension requires aggressive management, but should generally include an angiotensin-converting enzyme (ACE) inhibitor or angiotensin-receptor blockers (ARBs) (see Chapter 5). Liver cysts occasionally need resecting.

A recent placebo-controlled trial has suggested that treatment with the vasopressin receptor antagonist tolvaptan may lead to a slower rate of cyst growth and reduced rate of renal function loss in the short term.

### Hereditary nephritis (Alport's syndrome)

Hereditary nephritis is a group of rare genetic disorders that affects 2 in 100 000 people, and accounts for 3% of children and 0.2% of adults with ESKD in developed countries. It is caused by mutations in type IV collagen, which result in structurally defective glomerular (and other) basement membranes. Hereditary nephritis presents with hematuria and proteinuria, causes deafness and ocular changes, and in some individuals progresses to chronic kidney failure (CKD), but with a wide variation in phenotype.

**Pathophysiology.** There are three genetic forms of hereditary nephritis:
- mutations in the *COL4A5* gene causing X-linked Alport's syndrome (80% of patients)
- mutations in either *COL4A3* or *COL4A4* causing autosomal-recessive disease (15% of patients)
- mutations causing autosomal-dominant inheritance (5% of cases).

**Clinical features** are variable (Table 8.2). Males invariably progress to ESKD, while females, despite hematuria, generally maintain kidney function (15% may have CKD). Hematuria may be observed at birth. In adolescent boys, episodes of gross hematuria may be precipitated by upper respiratory infections. The absence of hematuria during the first 10 years of life makes it likely that a child will not be affected. The key pathological findings on kidney biopsy are seen by electron microscopy (thickening of the glomerular basement membrane, lamellation and electron-lucent areas).

*Other organ involvement.* About 50% of patients are deaf, males being more commonly affected than females. Deafness is usually progressive from birth onwards; in its early stages, the hearing deficit is detectable only by audiometry.

TABLE 8.2

**Clinical features of hereditary nephritis**

- Hematuria, albuminuria and hypertension
- Cochlear deafness
- Ocular abnormalities: anterior lenticonus and pigment changes in the perimacular region
- Platelet abnormalities (megathrombocytopenia)
- Prognosis: end-stage kidney disease in all affected males with X-linked disease, benign course in affected females

The most common ocular abnormalities are anterior lenticonus and/or pigment abnormalities of the macula. In lenticonus, the central portion of the lens protrudes into the anterior chamber, which causes progressive opacification of the lens leading to loss of visual acuity and progressive myopia. Lenticonus is usually associated with deafness and appears during the second to third decade of life. Pigment changes in the perimacular region consist of whitish or yellowish granulations surrounding the fovea. Hematologic defects (megathrombocytopenia) are rare.

**Diagnosis.** The differential diagnosis of hereditary nephritis includes various primary and secondary glomerular diseases causing hematuria, especially thin basement membrane disease and immunoglobulin (Ig)A nephropathy, and abnormalities of the urinary tract. The definitive diagnostic test is kidney biopsy with electron microscopy, and immunohistology showing the absence of specific collagen proteins. Skin biopsy and immunohistology can also be used, since the $\alpha5$ chains of type IV collagen are also found in the epidermal basement membrane.

Genetic analysis is the only reliable way to diagnose the carrier state in asymptomatic female members of affected families and to establish a prenatal diagnosis. However, the clinical usefulness of molecular genetic analysis is limited; it is time consuming and expensive and only identifies 50% of mutations. Thus, the most common approach still focuses on making a histological diagnosis, followed by screening family members by urinalysis and genetic counseling.

Recent work shows that some patients with thin basement membrane lesions have a heterozygous deficiency of either $\alpha3$ or $\alpha4$ type IV collagen chains. Although usually benign, some families show slow progression to CKD.

**Management.** No specific treatments are available. Priorities are management of hypertension, slowing the progression of CKD and prevention of complications. Ultimately, many patients progress to ESKD, requiring dialysis or transplantation. Transplant survival rates are similar to those for patients with other diagnoses (see Chapter 12). Anti-glomerular basement membrane nephritis involving the kidney allograft may occur in a recipient with hereditary nephritis, because an immune response develops to a hitherto unseen type IV collagen antigen; however, this is rare and affects only 3–4% of male transplant recipients.

Surgical repair of cataracts or repair of the anterior lenticonus is possible. Loss of hearing is likely to be permanent. Young men with Alport's syndrome should use hearing protection in noisy environments.

---

**Key points – inherited kidney disease**

- Autosomal-dominant polycystic kidney disease is a common inherited disease.
- Liver cysts are the most common extrarenal manifestation.
- Progression to end-stage kidney disease is slow, and does not occur in all patients.
- Alport's syndrome is an important but rare cause of hematuria.
- Deafness and eye abnormalities are common in men with Alport's syndrome.

---

**Key references**

Grantham JJ. Clinical practice. Autosomal dominant polycystic kidney disease. *N Engl J Med* 2008;359:1477–85.

Heidet L, Gubler MC. The renal lesions of Alport syndrome. *J Am Soc Nephrol* 2009;20:1210–5.

Pei Y. Practical genetics for autosomal dominant polycystic kidney disease. *Nephron Clin Pract* 2011;118:c19–30.

Torres VE, Harris PC. Autosomal dominant polycystic kidney disease: the last 3 years. *Kidney Int* 2009;76:149–68.

Urinary tract infection (UTI) is the presence of bacteria and white cells in the urine, together with symptoms; significant bacteriuria is defined as a urine culture yielding more than $10^5$ colony-forming units (CFU) of bacteria per mL of urine. Cystitis is inflammation of the bladder, which is most commonly (but not only) caused by infection. UTI is the second most common infection after respiratory infection and, in the elderly, is the most common source of Gram-negative bacteremia. However, UTI is generally a disease of sexually active females; 1 in 3 women will develop a UTI during her lifetime, and 20% have a recurrence. UTI is a leading cause of morbidity and healthcare expenditure; in the USA alone, UTI accounts for approximately 7 million visits per year to primary care providers and more than 1 million hospitalizations, and costs the US healthcare system in excess of $1 billion/year. In the UK, UTIs are the second largest single group of healthcare-associated infections and make up 20% of all hospital-acquired infections. In primary care, UTIs make up 1–3% of all practitioner consultations.

Also see Urinary tract infections and cystitis in *Fast Facts: Bladder Disorders*.

## Causes and risk factors

Most UTIs are caused by Gram-negative aerobic bacteria (Table 9.1). These bacteria are normally present in the colon and may enter the urethral opening from the skin around the anus and the vaginal introitus. Women may be more susceptible to UTI because their urethral opening is near the source of bacteria (i.e. anus, vagina) and their urethra is shorter, providing bacteria easier access to the bladder. In over 50% of patients, bacteria ascend further up the ureters to the kidneys.

Host factors predisposing to UTI are shown in Table 9.2. Factors influencing bacterial virulence are also important and include specific projecting hairlike structures called pili and fimbriae, which interact with the urothelium and enable the bacteria to adhere to the surface.

Sexual intercourse triggers UTI in some women for unknown reasons. Women who use a diaphragm develop infections more often, and condoms

TABLE 9.1

**Common causes of urinary tract infection**

| Source of infection | Organism | Incidence (%) |
|---|---|---|
| Community | Gram-negative | |
| | • *Escherichia coli* | 80 |
| | • *Klebsiella, Proteus, Enterobacter, Serratia* | 10 |
| | Gram-positive | |
| | • *Staphylococcus saprophyticus* | 8 |
| | • *Enterococci* | 2 |
| Hospital | Gram-negative | |
| | • *Escherichia coli* | 50 |
| | • *Klebsiella, Proteus, Enterobacter, Serratia* | 40 |
| | Gram-positive | |
| | • *Staphylococcus saprophyticus* and *S. aureus* | 8 |
| | • *Enterococcus faecalis* | 2 |
| | Yeasts | |
| | • *Candida, Blastomyces, Coccidiodes immitis* | < 5 |

TABLE 9.2

**Host factors predisposing to urinary tract infection**

| Premenopausal women | Postmenopausal women |
|---|---|
| • Sexual intercourse | • Previous UTI |
| • Spermicide cream | • Anatomic defects (e.g. incontinence, postvoid residual volume) |
| • Recent antibiotic use | |
| • Previous UTI | • Cystocele |
| • Maternal history of UTI | • Altered vaginal flora with estrogen deficiency |

UTI, urinary tract infection.

with spermicidal foam may allow the growth of *Escherichia coli* in the vagina, which may enter the urethra. Urinary catheterization can also cause UTIs by introducing bacteria into the urinary tract. In infants, bacteria from soiled diapers can enter the urethra and cause UTI. Other risk factors include bladder outlet obstruction (e.g. from kidney stones or benign prostatic hypertrophy), conditions that cause incomplete bladder emptying (e.g. spinal cord injury) and congenital abnormalities of the urinary tract (e.g. vesicoureteral reflux). In children under 10 years of age, 30–50% of UTIs are associated with vesicoureteral reflux and kidney scarring, which can lead to renal insufficiency if not treated.

## Diagnosis

The diagnosis of UTI requires a good history, urinalysis (with a Gram stain if indicated) and a clean-catch urine specimen for culture and sensitivity testing (Table 9.3). Urine culture may be unnecessary in a woman with a convincing history and pyuria on dipstick analysis.

TABLE 9.3

**Diagnosis of urinary tract infection**

| Technique | Feature identified |
|---|---|
| Urine dipstick | • Pyuria<br>• Hematuria<br>• Proteinuria |
| Urine sediment examination | • Leukocytes (upper limit of normal is 5 cells/high-power field)<br>• Erythrocytes (upper limit of normal is 5 cells/high-power field)<br>• Renal tubular epithelial cells<br>• Bacteria, yeast<br>• White-cell casts (suggestive of pyelonephritis) |
| Clean-catch urine for culture | • Positive culture |
| Imaging studies (ultrasound, CT scan of kidneys, ureter and bladder, or MRI) | • Indicated in all children (sometimes with a micturating cystourethrogram)<br>• Indicated in men with complicated UTI<br>• Indicated in women if response to treatment has been poor or recurrent episodes<br>• Indicated for any UTI associated with bacteremia or pyelonephritis |

CT, computerized tomography; MRI, magnetic resonance imaging; UTI, urinary tract infection.

## Treatment

Most patients respond rapidly to therapy. Structural abnormalities, such as prostatic hypertrophy or kidney calculi, require urologic referral. Hospitalization of patients with a UTI is unnecessary unless there is systemic toxicity and/or the patient requires intravenous antibiotic therapy. A 2008 Cochrane review suggested that drinking cranberry juice can be beneficial. Recommendations are for one cranberry tablet, 300–400 mg twice daily, or unsweetened juice, 250 mL or 8 oz three times daily. Drinking ample fluid also seems sensible. However, alkalinization of urine with potassium citrate remains unproven.

## UTI syndromes

UTI may be either uncomplicated or complicated. Uncomplicated UTI occurs in healthy (usually) women in the community. Complicated UTI occurs because of the presence of an underlying anatomic, functional or pharmacological factor that predisposes to persistent or recurrent infection, or treatment failure (Table 9.4). About one-third of all UTIs are complicated. The different categories, criteria for diagnosis and treatment of both complicated and uncomplicated UTIs are summarized in Table 9.5.

**Acute cystitis in young women** is the most common category of UTI and occurs in young, sexually active women. Causative factors may include sexual activity itself and the use of diaphragms and spermicides. While traditionally the diagnosis of UTI is based on the presence of significant bacteriuria, one-third or more of symptomatic women with uncomplicated cystitis have less than $10^5$ CFU/mL of urine, and a convincing history with pyuria by dipstick has a high predictive value without the need for urine culture.

TABLE 9.4

**Clinical complications of urinary tract infection**

- Hemorrhagic cystitis
- Abscess of the bladder wall (pyocystosis)
- Papillary necrosis
- Chronic pyelonephritis
- Kidney abscess
- Kidney failure
- Septic shock

TABLE 9.5

## Diagnosis and treatment of urinary tract infections in adults

| Diagnosis | Treatment |
| --- | --- |
| **Acute uncomplicated cystitis** | |
| Clinical diagnosis or urine culture (> $10^2$ CFU/mL) | See Tables 9.6 and 9.7 |
| **Recurrent cystitis in young women** | |
| Urine culture (> $10^2$–$10^6$ CFU/mL) | • Change contraception method<br>• Treat as for acute uncomplicated cystitis (see Tables 9.6 and 9.7)<br>• Consider prophylaxis for 6 months |
| **Postcoital urinary tract infection** | |
| History | • Consider single-dose, postcoital antibiotic prophylaxis using same drugs and doses as for recurrent cystitis prophylaxis (above) |
| **UTI in adult male** | |
| Urine culture (> $10^3$ CFU/mL) | • Consider all UTIs in men complicated, including the possibility that infection has ascended to the kidneys<br>• Assume there is infection of the upper urinary tract<br>• Treat for 10–14 days with outpatient antibiotic regimen<br>• Adjust treatment plan if antibiotic sensitivity testing demonstrates a resistant organism |
| **Acute pyelonephritis** | |
| History and urine culture (> $10^6$ CFU/mL) | • Treat for 7–14 days orally, or intravenously initially if unwell |
| **Asymptomatic bacteriuria in pregnancy** | |
| Isolation of the same bacterial strain in two consecutive voided specimens (> $10^5$ CFU/mL) | • Treat asymptomatic bacteriuria and cystitis with oral antibiotics<br>• Avoid quinolones |
| **Catheter-associated infection** | |
| Urine culture (> $10^5$ CFU/mL) | • Remove catheter if possible<br>• Treat with antibiotics for 7–10 days according to sensitivity |

* The exact number of bacteria in a urine culture needed to define UTI in men is controversial: positive results are seen with > 1000 CFU/mL, much lower than the threshold for women, but most clinicians accept > 10 000 CFU/mL.
CFU, colony-forming units.

The symptoms of cystitis usually have a sudden onset and include urinary frequency, urgency and burning or painful voiding of small volumes of urine. Nocturia with suprapubic or low back pain is common. The urine is often turbid, and gross hematuria occurs in about 30% of patients. This is not a systemic infection, and patients should not be febrile or develop a raised erythrocyte sedimentation rate (ESR) or C-reactive protein. Uncomplicated cystitis is most commonly caused by *E. coli* and is easily treated with antibiotics; 3-day courses may be better than single doses or 7-day courses (Table 9.6).

TABLE 9.6

**Guidelines and regimens for the treatment of urinary tract infections in women**

- Treat uncomplicated acute bacterial cystitis in all women (including ≥ 65 years old) with antibiotics (level A), with a treatment regimen as follows:

| Drug/dose | Adverse events |
|---|---|
| Trimethoprim, 160 mg, and sulfamethoxazole, 800 mg, bd for 3 days (one tablet) | Fever, rash, photosensitivity, neutropenia, thrombocytopenia, anorexia, nausea and vomiting, pruritus, headache, urticaria, Stevens–Johnson syndrome, toxic epidermal necrosis |
| Trimethoprim, 100 mg, bd for 3 days | Rash, pruritus, photosensitivity, exfoliative dermatitis, Stevens–Johnson syndrome, toxic epidermal necrosis, aseptic meningitis |
| Ciprofloxacin, 250 mg, bd for 3 days | Rash, confusion, seizures, restlessness, headache, severe hypersensitivity, hypoglycemia, hyperglycemia, Achilles tendon rupture (in patients > 60 years) |
| Levofloxacin, 250 mg, od for 3 days | Same as for ciprofloxacin |
| Norfloxacin, 400 mg, bd for 3 days | Same as for ciprofloxacin |
| Gatifloxacin, 200 mg, od for 3 days | Same as for ciprofloxacin |

CONTINUED

TABLE 9.6 (CONTINUED)

| | |
|---|---|
| Nitrofurantoin macrocrystals, 50–100 mg, qd for 7 days | Anorexia, nausea, vomiting, hypersensitivity, peripheral neuropathy, hepatitis, hemolytic anemia, pulmonary reactions |
| Nitrofurantoin monohydrate crystals, 100 mg, bd for 7 days | Same as for nitrofurantoin macrocrystals |
| Fosfomycin tromethamine, 3 g (powder) single dose | Diarrhea, nausea, vomiting, rash, hypersensitivity |

- Complete 14 days of antimicrobial therapy in all cases of acute pyelonephritis (inpatient and outpatient) (level A)
- Change antibiotic class if resistance rates > 15–20% (level A)
- No need to screen, or treat, asymptomatic bacteriuria in non-pregnant, pre-menopausal women (level A)
- No need for urine culture before treatment of symptomatic lower UTI with pyuria or bacteriuria (level B)
- The antimicrobials listed above are more effective than beta-lactams (e.g. first-generation cephalosporins and amoxicillin) in the treatment of acute uncomplicated cystitis (level C)
- Decrease urine count to CFU $10^2$–$10^4$/mL in symptomatic patients to improve sensitivity without significantly compromising specificity (level C)

Level A – good, consistent evidence; level B – limited, inconsistent evidence; level C – consensus, expert opinion evidence. bd, twice daily; od, once daily; qd, four times daily.
Adapted from American College of Obstetricians and Gynecologists (ACOG). *Practice Bulletin* 2008;91:10.

**Recurrent cystitis in young women.** Up to 20% of young women with acute cystitis develop recurrent UTIs. Hematuria and pyuria are almost always present. It is important to perform a urine culture to differentiate between relapse (infection with the same organism) and recurrence (infection with different organisms). Multiple infections caused by the same organism require longer courses of antibiotics and possibly further diagnostic tests. In contrast, infections caused by different organisms are generally not associated with underlying anatomic abnormalities and do not require further investigation of the genitourinary tract. A negative urinalysis or Gram stain does not exclude cystitis in women with low bacterial counts.

Women who have more than three recurrences of UTI documented by urine culture within 1 year can be managed by either self-treatment of the acute episode, postcoital prophylaxis (if an association with sexual intercourse is established) or continuous daily prophylaxis (see Table 9.5). This approach decreases the significant morbidity associated with recurrent UTIs and is not associated with induction of antibiotic resistance in the organisms. However, stopping antibiotic prophylaxis is associated with recurrence in over 50% of patients.

**Acute cystitis in young men** is most commonly associated with underlying urologic abnormalities. In younger men, however, UTI may result from unprotected anal intercourse, an uncircumcised penis, unprotected intercourse with a woman whose vagina is colonized with uropathogens and in those men with HIV infection and a CD4+ T-cell count below 200/µL. The commonest urologic abnormalities that predispose to UTI are prostatic disease and outlet obstruction (see Chapter 11) and urinary tract instrumentation.

A diagnosis of UTI can be made with a high degree of sensitivity and specificity if the patient has symptoms of UTI and bacteriuria of more than $10^3$ CFU/mL of urine. Treatment should be given for 10–14 days (see Table 9.5), and for as long as 6–12 weeks in acute prostatitis. In complicated UTI, further diagnostic investigations should be performed, but no further action may be necessary in younger men who respond rapidly to treatment. Chronic prostatitis may be more occult and present only as recurrent bacteriuria, low-grade fever or back discomfort. It is the commonest cause of recurrent UTI in men.

**Acute urethritis** usually presents with dysuria and urethral discharge, and is caused by gonococci, *Chlamydia* or *Ureaplasma* (non-specific urethritis). It is often associated with vaginal discharge and dyspareunia. Midstream urine does not contain blood on urinalysis.

**Urethral syndrome** occurs in women complaining of recurrent dysuria and frequency, but with sterile urine or low bacterial counts that have not responded to antibiotics. Vaginitis is found in 30% of these women (*Candida*, *Trichomonas* or non-specific), but the cause is unknown in the remainder.

**Acute pyelonephritis** is bacterial infection of the kidney parenchyma. In men, pyelonephritis does not usually occur in the absence of underlying urologic abnormalities, whereas in women it may occur in association with, or as a consequence of, acute cystitis even in the absence of predisposing factors. Occasionally, bacterial infection is not ascending, but occurs by hematogenous spread of a virulent bacterial strain (e.g. *Salmonella, Staphylococcus aureus*). In some patients, pyelonephritis may present with mild cystitis-like symptoms accompanied by back pain, while in others, a more severe illness occurs characterized by fever, chills, hypotension and severe back pain with or without symptoms of acute cystitis.

In most cases, acute pyelonephritis is caused by specific uropathogenic strains of *E. coli* that possess adhesins. These strains are able to ascend the urinary tract and adhere to renal tubular cells. Patients have elevated C-reactive protein and white cell counts, pyuria and, in 20%, positive blood cultures. The urine may contain white-cell casts, but proteinuria is minimal. The commonest organisms are *E. coli*, staphylococci, enterococci, and *Klebsiella*. The differential diagnosis includes appendicitis, urolithiasis, pelvic inflammatory disease, ectopic pregnancy and ruptured ovarian cyst.

For patients with a mild presentation, oral therapy is sufficient (see Table 9.5). For patients with more severe symptoms or with evidence of bacteremia, empiric parenteral antibiotic therapy is recommended for at least the first 1–3 days: a third-generation cephalosporin, aztreonam, a broad-spectrum penicillin, a quinolone, an aminoglycoside or trimethoprim–sulfamethoxazole, followed by oral therapy; in this case, treatment should be given for a minimum of 2 weeks.

**Chronic pyelonephritis** is a term usually reserved for recurrent episodes of pyelonephritis in the presence of vesicoureteric reflux in children, but can occur in other circumstances. Kidney parenchymal scarring occurs and can lead to progressive kidney failure.

**Asymptomatic bacteriuria** is bacteriuria of more than $10^5$ CFU/mL of urine in asymptomatic individuals. Treatment is warranted only in certain circumstances (Table 9.7). Although up to 40% of the elderly have asymptomatic bacteriuria, it is unclear whether treatment is beneficial in reducing complications or mortality.

Between 2–10% of pregnancies are complicated by UTI; if left untreated, 25–30% of the women affected will develop pyelonephritis.

TABLE 9.7

**Indications for treatment of asymptomatic bacteriuria**

- Pregnancy, particularly in third trimester
- Predisposition to renal disease (e.g. polycystic kidney disease)
- Immunocompromised patient (e.g. kidney transplant)
- Patients requiring urologic manipulation
- Patients with anatomic or urologic abnormalities of the urinary tract

Pregnancies that are complicated by pyelonephritis have been associated with low-birth-weight and premature infants. Thus, pregnant women should be screened for bacteriuria by urine culture at 12–16 weeks of gestation. Bacteriuria of more than $10^5$ CFU/mL of urine is considered significant. Pregnant women with asymptomatic bacteriuria should be treated with a 3–7-day course of antibiotics (see Table 9.5), and the urine should subsequently be cultured to ensure cure and to avoid relapse. As *E. coli* is now commonly resistant to ampicillin, amoxicillin and cefalexin, treatment should be based on the results of susceptibility tests. Nitrofurantoin or trimethoprim–sulfamethoxazole may be used, but in the third trimester sulfonamides compete with bilirubin binding in the newborn.

Most pregnant women with pyelonephritis should be hospitalized. They should receive intravenous antibiotic therapy initially, then oral treatment for 14 days, followed by nightly suppressive therapy until delivery. Ceftriaxone is a suitable agent for inpatient treatment, but the fluoroquinolones should be avoided in pregnancy.

**Catheter-associated urinary tract infection.** The risk of bacteriuria is approximately 5% per day in patients with an indwelling urinary catheter. Therefore, bacteriuria is inevitable in patients undergoing long-term catheterization. Catheter-associated UTIs account for 40% of all nosocomial infections and are the most common source of Gram-negative bacteremia in hospitalized patients. The bacterial distribution reflects the nosocomial origin of the infections, which are often polymicrobial because many of the pathogens are acquired exogenously via manipulation of the catheter. Symptomatic bacteriuria in a patient with an indwelling catheter should be treated with antibiotics that cover potential nosocomial uropathogens (see Table 9.5). Patients with mild-to-moderate infections may be treated with an oral quinolone, usually for 10–14 days. Parenteral antibiotic therapy may be necessary for patients with severe infections or patients who are unable to tolerate oral medication.

Treatment is not recommended for catheterized patients who have asymptomatic bacteriuria, with the exception of patients who are immunosuppressed after organ transplantation, patients at risk for bacterial endocarditis and patients who are about to undergo urinary tract instrumentation.

## Key points – urinary tract infection

- Uncomplicated cystitis in women, diagnosed by history and pyuria, can be treated empirically with short courses of antibiotics.
- Recurrent cystitis in women may require longer courses of, or prophylactic, antibiotics.
- Cystitis in men generally requires a formal urologic assessment.
- Pyelonephritis usually requires intravenous antibiotics as initial treatment.

## Key references

American College of Obstetricians and Gynecologists (ACOG) 2008. *Treatment of urinary tract infections in nonpregnant women.* http://guideline.gov/summary/summary.aspx?doc_id=12628, last accessed 09 May 2013.

Chenoweth CE, Saint S. Urinary tract infections. *Infect Dis Clin North Am* 2011;25:103–15.

Enzler MJ, Berbari E, Osmon DR. Antimicrobial prophylaxis in adults. *Mayo Clin Proc* 2011;86:686–701.

Jepson RG, Craig JC. Cranberries for preventing urinary tract infections. *Conchrane Database Syst Rev* 2008(1):CD001321.

Lane DR, Takhar SS. Diagnosis and management of urinary tract infection and pyelonephritis. *Emerg Med Clin North Am* 2011;29: 539–52.

Slack A, Newman DK, Wein AJ. *Fast Facts: Bladder Disorders*, 2nd edn. Oxford: Health Press, 2011.

Kidney stones are a common cause of morbidity in the Western world, affecting 10–20% of the population during their lifetime and leading to hospitalization for 1 in 1000 of the general population each year. Over 80% of kidney stones occur in white men; they are much rarer in women and black people. The peak age of onset for kidney stone formation is 20–30 years, and the recurrence rate is high – up to 50% within 5 years.

There are four main types of kidney stones (Table 10.1).

- The most common stones contain calcium salts, and may be calcium oxalate, calcium phosphate or a mixture of both.
- Magnesium ammonium phosphate stones (struvite stones) mostly occur in association with an underlying urease-splitting bacterial infection of the urinary tract (e.g. Proteus). These stones often recur and are most often seen in patients with an associated anatomic abnormality.
- Pure uric acid stones usually occur in the context of hyperuricemia among patients with a gouty diathesis or a hematologic malignancy. Uric acid stones have a high recurrence rate.
- Cystine stones are extremely rare and occur in patients with cystinuria, which is an autosomal defect in the transport of the amino acids cystine, ornithine, lysine and arginine in the kidney and intestine.

TABLE 10.1

**Incidence of different types of kidney stone**

| Type of stone | Incidence (%) |
| --- | --- |
| Calcium | 70–80 |
| • calcium oxalate | 70 |
| • calcium phosphate | < 5 |
| • mixed calcium oxalate/phosphate | < 5 |
| Magnesium ammonium phosphate (struvite) | 10–20 |
| Uric acid | 5–10 |
| Cystine | < 1 |

Rarely, drugs can crystallize in the urine and form stones (e.g. indinavir, triamterene, aciclovir).

## Risk factors

The most important risk factors for kidney stones are the supersaturation of urine with calcium oxalate and/or uric acid, and the pH of the urine (Table 10.2); however, other underlying risk factors are not completely understood. Reduced levels or absence of urinary inhibitors of stone formation, such as citrate, also favor stone formation. Urinary infection with a urease-splitting organism is a key factor in struvite stone formation.

TABLE 10.2

**Risk factors for kidney stone formation**

| Risk factor | Example |
| --- | --- |
| Supersaturation of urine with solute | • Hypercalciuria<br>• Hyperoxaluria |
| Inadequate inhibition of stone formation | • Hypocitraturia<br>• Reduced urinary osteopontin |
| Anatomic abnormalities | • Pyelocalyceal diverticula<br>• Pelviureteric junction obstruction<br>• Horseshoe kidney |
| Diet | • High protein intake, excess sodium, low urine volume (especially in stone-belt area in southeastern USA and Middle East) |
| Urinary pH | • Urinary tract infection caused by urease-splitting organism promotes alkaline urine and struvite stone formation<br>• Acid urine favors formation of uric acid and cystine stones |
| Medication | • Acetazolamide increases urine pH and calcium excretion<br>• Triamterene crystallizes in urine and forms a nidus for stone formation<br>• Vitamin C<br>• Calcium and vitamin D<br>• Theophylline |

## Pathophysiology

**Calcium stone disease.** The most common stones are calcium oxalate stones rather than pure calcium phosphate. The major cause of calcium stone formation is excessive urinary excretion of calcium (hypercalciuria), with or without hypercalcemia. The most common cause of hypercalcemia is primary hyperparathyroidism. Hypercalciuria without hypercalcemia is observed in 60% of patients with calcium stones. The primary abnormality appears to be impairment in renal tubular resorption of calcium, but it also reflects increased absorption of dietary calcium and excessive bone resorption. Other less common etiologies include hyperuricosuria in about 10% of patients, hyperoxaluria, hypocitraturia and medullary sponge kidney.

**Non-calcareous stone disease.** The most common type of non-calcareous stones are struvite stones, which are also termed 'infection' stones, because they are usually associated with urinary tract infection (UTI) by a urea-splitting organism. Bacterial urease degrades urea into ammonia (and subsequently ammonium), resulting in alkaline urine, which favors the formation of triphosphate ions and reduces the solubility of struvite. Uric acid stone formation is also critically dependent on the urinary pH.

A urinary pH lower than the dissociation constant for uric acid (pH 5.5) and/or the presence of hyperuricosuria play major roles in uric acid stone formation. Chronic diarrheal syndromes, such as ulcerative colitis and Crohn's disease, and jejunoileal bypass surgery are associated with reduced urinary pH and thus a greater propensity for uric acid stone formation. Hyperuricosuria is most frequently observed in states of purine overproduction, such as myeloproliferative states and glycogen storage diseases.

## Clinical features

Clinical presentation varies depending on the location, size and number of stones. The most common presentation is renal colic, which is the sudden onset of severe pain caused by the presence of an obstructing kidney or ureteral stone. Renal colic is typically spasmodic, lasts several minutes, is localized to the flank and radiates down to the groin, accompanied by nausea and vomiting. It often occurs in the middle of the night or early morning while the patient is sedentary, and its severity has been described as akin to or worse than childbirth. On the other hand, larger stones may present with painless obstruction or back pain. Stones that reach the ureterovesical junction often present with renal colic accompanied by urgency and frequency. Stones located in the kidney calyces may be completely asymptomatic. Patients with renal colic are often writhing in excruciating pain and restless. The presence of fever usually heralds an accompanying UTI. Otherwise, the physical examination may be completely unremarkable.

## Diagnosis

Laboratory evaluation should include a complete blood count, blood chemistry including measurement of blood urea nitrogen (BUN or serum urea) and creatinine, and urinalysis (Table 10.3). The presence of a UTI, particularly with pyelonephritis, will be associated with leukocytosis. An elevated BUN and creatinine would suggest dehydration and/or the presence of an obstructing stone in a patient with a single kidney, or

TABLE 10.3

**Diagnosis of kidney stones**

**Identify the number, size and location of stones**
- Radiopaque stones can be seen on a plain abdominal radiograph of the kidneys, ureters and bladder
- Radiolucent stones can be detected by ultrasound, CT or intravenous pyelography
- Imaging will also detect evidence of kidney outflow obstruction

**Analysis of the chemical composition of the stone**
- Strain urine (use a coffee filter paper)
- Send stone to a specialist laboratory for stone analysis

**Metabolic investigations**
- Urinalysis, urine pH and urine culture
- Blood chemistry, including blood urea nitrogen (serum urea), creatinine, calcium, electrolytes, bicarbonate and complete blood count
- 24-hour urine collection for volume, pH, calcium, phosphorus, sodium, uric acid, oxalate, citrate, cystine and creatinine (collect at least two specimens to account for variability)

bilateral obstructing stones. Hematuria and pyuria are usually present. Assessment of urine pH is critical, because acid urine with a radiolucent stone suggests a uric acid stone, while an alkaline urine (pH > 8.0) suggests infection with a urease-splitting organism (e.g. *Proteus*, *Pseudomonas*, *Klebsiella*). Imaging should include a radiograph of the kidney, ureters and bladder, and an ultrasound or a non-contrast CT scan (Figure 10.1).

## Management

Initially, management is directed towards optimal pain control, hydration and urologic consultation for potential removal of an obstructing stone, and subsequently to the underlying predisposing factors and prevention of further episodes. Medical management of a non-obstructing stone requires increasing fluid intake to generate a urine output of more than 2 liters/day, dietary modification and treatment targeted at changing urinary pH (Tables 10.4 and 10.5). Low-calcium diets are to be avoided.

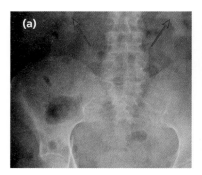 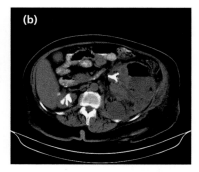

**Figure 10.1** (a) Plain abdominal radiograph showing bilateral staghorn calculi; (b) CT scan of bilateral staghorn calculi and a secondary left kidney abscess.

TABLE 10.4

**Dietary modifications for long-term management of kidney stones**

- **High fluid intake:** at least 10 glasses/day
- **Sodium restriction:** avoid salty foods, adding salt to meals, prepared meals
- **Oxalate restriction:** avoid nuts, spinach, chocolate, tea and vitamin C
- **Purine reduction:** reduce meat protein intake especially
- **High citrate intake:** increase intake of citrus fruits

TABLE 10.5

**Management of kidney stone disease**

| Abnormality | Management |
| --- | --- |
| **Calcium oxalate** | |
| Hyperoxaluria | • Reduce oxalate intake (rhubarb, spinach, beetroot, chocolate, peanuts, strawberries, tea, wheat bran)<br>• If ileal disease is present, give oral calcium supplement and cholestyramine |
| Hyperuricosuria | • Allopurinol, 100–600 mg/day<br>• Reduce purine intake (proteins)<br>• Alkalinize urine to pH > 6.5 with sodium bicarbonate, 60–100 mmol/day |
| **Calcium phosphate** | |
| Hypercalciuria | • As above<br>• Treat underlying disorder (e.g. hyperparathyroidism, renal tubular acidosis)<br>• Stop acetazolamide<br>• Potassium bicarbonate or citrate |
| **Magnesium ammonium phosphate (struvite)** | |
| Infection | • Remove all stone material followed by prolonged antibiotics to ensure urine sterility<br>• If stones remain, prolong suppressive antibiotics<br>• Urease inhibitor (acetohydroxamine) as adjunctive therapy |
| **Uric acid** | |
| Hyperuricemia | • Increase hydration (urine output > 2 L/day)<br>• Alkalinize urine with potassium citrate<br>• Reduce meat intake<br>• Allopurinol, 100–600 mg/day<br>• Avoid uricosuric agents |
| **Cystine** | |
| Cystinuria | • Increase hydration (urine output > 2 L/day)<br>• Reduce methionine-rich protein in diet<br>• Raise urine pH to > 6.5 with sodium bicarbonate<br>• Sulfahydryl-containing agent, such as penicillamine, 1–2 g/day, or tiopronin, 800 mg/day, but side effects are common |

**Surgical management** depends on the size, location and number of stones (Table 10.6). Indications for urologic surgery are:

- stones more than 5 mm in diameter
- stones impacted for more than 24 hours
- evidence of significant obstruction
- evidence of infection.

Obstruction may require percutaneous nephrostomy. Surgical options include extracorporeal shock-wave lithotripsy (ESWL) and stone removal (percutaneous or transurethral). Rules of thumb are that cystine and calcium oxalate monohydrate stones are generally poorly broken up by ESWL, while calcium oxalate, struvite and uric acid stones are usually amenable to ESWL, as well as to removal by either the percutaneous or transurethral route, depending on the size and location of the stones.

TABLE 10.6

**Surgical management of kidney stones**

| Location and size of stone | Management |
|---|---|
| **Kidney** | |
| < 0.5 cm, asymptomatic | Observe |
| 0.5–2 cm | Consider ESWL |
| > 2 cm or lower pole and > 1 cm | Percutaneous approach or ESWL |
| **Ureter** | |
| < 0.5 cm | Conservative management – may pass spontaneously |
| > 0.5 cm or not progressing | Proximal – push back and then ESWL (or PCNL) |
| | Distal – ESWL or ureteroscopic removal |

ESWL, extracorporeal shock-wave lithotripsy; PCNL, percutaneous nephrolithotomy.

## Key points – kidney stones

- Kidney stones are common and are most often associated with hypercalciuria.
- Stones can be asymptomatic or cause a variety of clinical problems.
- Stones may require surgical intervention, but recurrence after surgery is common.
- High fluid intake and a low-salt and low-oxalate diet are the mainstays of management.
- Low-calcium diets should be avoided.
- Thiazide diuretics and potassium citrate are used in some patients.

## Key references

Schade GR, Faerber GJ. Urinary tract stones. *Prim Care* 2010;37:565–81, ix.

Schissel BL, Johnson BK. Renal stones: evolving epidemiology and management. *Pediatr Emerg Care* 2011;27:676–81.

Singh SK, Agarwal MM, Sharma S. Medical therapy for calculus disease. *BJU Int* 2011;107:356–68.

Taylor JC, Gauer R, Rideout S. Clinical inquiries. Ureteral calculi: what should you consider before intervening? *J Fam Pract* 2011;60:232–3.

## Urinary tract obstruction

Urinary tract obstruction or obstructive uropathy is defined as complete or partial obstruction of the flow of urine at any level of the urinary tract from the kidneys to the urethral meatus. Urinary tract obstruction is a relatively common cause of community-acquired acute kidney injury (AKI) (10% of cases) with an incidence of 23 cases per million population. Urinary tract obstruction has a bimodal age distribution, and is common in children and the elderly (> 60 years of age). In children, congenital abnormalities of the urinary tract are particularly common, and include pelviureteric junction obstruction and vesicoureteric junction obstruction, such as an ectopic ureter, ureterocele or posterior urethral valves. In adults, the commonest causes are benign prostatic hyperplasia (BPH) in men and pelvic malignancies in women.

**Causes.** Urinary tract obstruction can be classified according to cause (congenital versus acquired), duration (acute versus chronic), degree (partial versus complete) and location (upper versus lower urinary tract). Major causes are summarized in Table 11.1. The most common mechanical cause is BPH (see *Fast Facts: Benign Prostatic Hyperplasia*). Common causes of functional bladder outlet obstruction include neurogenic bladders, detrusor sphincter dyssynergia and iatrogenic medical intervention, such as the use of anticholinergic drugs.

**Pathophysiology.** Three main points of physiological narrowing of the urinary tract present a high risk for obstruction: the pelviureteric junction, the crossing of the ureter over the common iliac vessels at the pelvic brim and the vesicoureteric junction (Figure 11.1). The functional effects of urinary tract obstruction are influenced by the level, severity and duration of obstruction. Short-term complete infravesical obstruction is invariably associated with AKI together with an enlarged bladder, hydroureter and hydronephrosis. These abnormalities are reversible and rarely associated with long-term sequelae if diagnosed and treated early. Long-term complete infravesical obstruction may result in

TABLE 11.1

**Causes of urinary tract obstruction**

| Intrinsic | Extrinsic |
|---|---|
| *Intraluminal causes* | *Originating in the reproductive system* |
| • Intratubular deposition of crystals (uric acid, sulfates) | • Prostate – benign hyperplasia, cancer |
| • Stones | • Uterus – pregnancy, tumors, prolapse, endometriosis |
| • Papillary tissue | • Ovary – abscess, tumor, cysts |
| • Blood clots | *Originating in the vascular system* |
| *Intramural functional causes* | • Aneurysms (aorta, iliac vessels) |
| • Ureter (ureteropelvic or ureterovesical dysfunction) | • Aberrant arteries (pelviureteric junction) |
| • Bladder (neurogenic) – spinal cord defect or trauma, diabetes, multiple sclerosis, Parkinson's disease, cerebrovascular accidents, drugs | • Venous (ovarian veins, retrocaval ureter) |
| | *Originating in the gastrointestinal tract* |
| | • Crohn's disease |
| • Bladder neck dysfunction | • Pancreatitis |
| *Intramural anatomic causes* | • Appendicitis |
| • Tumors | • Tumors |
| • Infection | *Originating in the retroperitoneal space* |
| • Granuloma | • Inflammation |
| • Strictures | • Fibrosis |
| | • Tumors |
| | • Hematomas |

AKI or subacute kidney failure coupled with structural changes that are often irreversible.

Obstruction to outflow from the bladder leads to hypertrophied muscle and marked trabeculation of the bladder wall, mucosal diverticula and, ultimately, detrusor muscle decompensation. Progressive back-pressure on the ureter and kidneys results in hydroureteronephrosis. Increased intrarenal pressure precipitates a reduction in renal blood flow, progressive ischemia, compression of the papillae, decreased glomerular filtration rate (GFR) and loss of parenchyma secondary to loss of

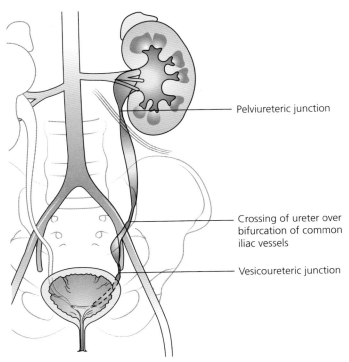

Pelviureteric junction

Crossing of ureter over
bifurcation of common
iliac vessels

Vesicoureteric junction

**Figure 11.1** The three main points of physiological narrowing of the urinary
tract – the pelviureteric junction, the crossing of the ureter over the common
iliac vessels at the pelvic brim and the vesicoureteric junction – present a high
risk for obstruction.

nephrons. Angiotensin II plays a pivotal role in this process, driving
inflammatory and profibrotic changes. The result of this heightened
cytokine activity is progressive irreversible kidney fibrosis.

**Clinical features.** The level of obstruction and its duration governs the
clinical presentation of urinary tract obstruction (Table 11.2). If the
obstruction is complicated by urinary tract infection (UTI) then symptoms
associated with the infection are also usually present (see Chapter 9).

Since lower tract obstruction in men is commonly due to prostatic
enlargement, a digital rectal examination is essential. In women, a
thorough pelvic examination is necessary to detect pelvic malignancies.

TABLE 11.2

**Clinical presentation of urinary tract obstruction**

Acute upper tract obstruction
- Flank pain
- Palpable enlarged kidney

Lower urinary tract obstruction
- Voiding difficulty
- Hesitancy
- Dribbling
- Inadequate bladder emptying

Chronic obstruction
- Symptoms and signs of chronic kidney failure (nausea, anorexia, weight loss, pruritus)

Chronic lower tract obstruction
- Urinary urgency
- Urge incontinence
- Bladder enlargement

**Diagnosis.** Urinary tract obstruction should be sought in any individual who presents with kidney failure of unknown cause. The history and physical examination are often crucial. Sudden onset of complete anuria is highly suggestive of urinary tract obstruction, and ultrasound examination is the preferred diagnostic investigation.

The finding of hydronephrosis in association with back-pressure changes in the kidney parenchyma is central to the diagnosis. However, hydronephrosis is not always caused by obstruction. For example, vesicoureteric reflux, papillary necrosis, brisk diuresis in nephrogenic diabetes insipidus and pregnancy may cause calyceal dilatation in the absence of obstruction. Hydronephrosis should be categorized as either obstructive or non-obstructive. With obstructive hydronephrosis, the degree of dilatation of the pelvicalyceal system may be an insensitive

121

indicator of the severity of obstruction. Some patients with acute complete obstruction may initially have mild or no hydronephrosis, because of the brief duration of the obstruction, low urine production or external compression from a retroperitoneal process. Thus, a normal ultrasound examination does not exclude obstruction.

In acute obstruction, the kidney cortex is intact, whereas chronic obstruction usually leads to marked thinning of the cortex. Failure to visualize the proximal ureter suggests obstruction at the pelviureteric junction, whereas a dilated ureter indicates an obstruction downstream, often at the level of the bladder. A large postvoid bladder indicates urinary retention, often as a result of prostatic enlargement, whereas an empty bladder with dilatation of the distal ureters suggests obstruction at the bladder inlet. Therefore, it is essential to examine the entire urinary tract when hydronephrosis is present.

Once a diagnosis of urinary obstruction has been made, further investigations are necessary to establish the underlying cause (Table 11.3, Figure 11.2). Contrast medium for intravenous urography or CT may lead to kidney dysfunction in patients with existing renal impairment and should be administered with caution. In most circumstances, after kidney ultrasonography, a CT scan followed by either antegrade or retrograde pyelography is the best approach. Assessment of lower tract obstruction to distinguish functional from mechanical causes may include uroflowmetry (to measure the speed of urine flow), postvoid residual urine measurement (to determine the amount of urine left in the bladder after urination) and filling cystometry (to determine the presence of uninhibited detrusor contractions).

**Treatment.** Most patients should be referred for urologic evaluation, because untreated obstruction may result in irreversible parenchymal kidney injury. Immediate referral is particularly important if there is:

- complete obstruction
- obstruction in a solitary kidney
- associated sepsis
- acute kidney injury
- uncontrolled colic and/or pain.

Obstruction coexisting with infection should be considered a urologic emergency and requires immediate relief with a Foley catheter, ureteral

TABLE 11.3

**Investigation of urinary tract obstruction**

### Urine

- Urinalysis
- Urine culture
- Urine cytology

### Blood

- Kidney function (blood urea nitrogen [serum urea] and creatinine)
- Prostate-specific antigen
- Serum tumor markers (CA-125)

### Imaging

- Postvoid residual urine
- Kidney ultrasonography
- Pelvic transvaginal ultrasonography
- Prostate ultrasonography
- Intravenous excretory urography
- Urethrocystoscopy (also called cystourethroscopy)

### Assessment of function

- Uroflowmetry
- Filling cystometry (also called cystometrography)

stent or percutaneous nephrostomy tube, and broad-spectrum antibiotics. In patients with partial obstruction, particularly in the setting of infection, initial management with analgesia and antibiotics is reasonable until a full evaluation can be completed. Colic secondary to urinary obstruction can be severe and is best managed with opioid analgesics, such as morphine sulfate, oxycodone and hydrocodone. Non-steroidal anti-inflammatory drugs (NSAIDs) or cyclo-oxygenase 2 inhibitors should be avoided if possible, because they may exacerbate or precipitate AKI. Antibiotic prophylaxis (e.g. trimethoprim, trimethoprim–sulfamethoxazole, cefalexin) should be initiated to cover common urinary pathogens.

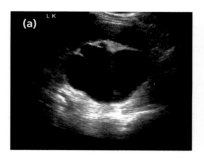
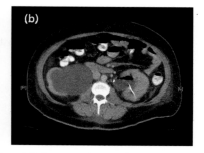

**Figure 11.2** Imaging renal tract obstruction. (a) Ultrasound scan of an obstructed kidney; (b) CT scan showing bilateral obstruction, a chronically obstructed right kidney with thin cortex and gross hydronephrosis, and mild dilatation of the left kidney, with nephrostomy tube in situ.

Surgical management may be temporary; for example, relieving the obstruction using a Foley catheter, ureteral stent or percutaneous nephrostomy tube. More definitive surgical intervention will depend on the cause, type and duration of obstruction.

## Tumors of the urinary tract

Tumors of the urinary tract can involve the kidney, ureters, bladder, prostate or urethra. Only tumors of the kidney are discussed here. For further information see *Fast Facts: Bladder Cancer* and *Fast Facts: Prostate Cancer*.

## Benign kidney tumors

There are broadly four categories of benign kidney tumor: mesenchymal, mixed epithelial and mesenchymal, renal cell, and metanephric (Table 11.4).

**Mesenchymal tumors.** Angiomyolipoma (AML) is the most common benign mesenchymal neoplasm, and is considered by some to be the most common benign renal tumor. It is composed of blood vessels, smooth muscle and adipose tissue. AML may occur spontaneously or in association with tuberous sclerosis complex, an autosomal dominant genetic disorder. Nearly 80% of patients with tuberous sclerosis will ultimately develop AMLs; these are typically multicentric and usually affect both kidneys. Spontaneous AMLs have a female preponderance and are usually solitary and symptomatic. Solitary AMLs may become very large and lead to pain, progressive kidney failure and hemorrhage within

TABLE 11.4

**World Health Organization histological classification of benign renal tumors**

| Renal cell tumors | Metanephric tumors |
|---|---|
| • Oncocytoma | • Metanephric adenoma |
| • Papillary adenoma | • Metanephric adenofibroma |
| | • Metanephric stromal tumor |
| **Mesenchymal tumors** | |
| • Angiomyolipoma | **Mixed epithelial and mesenchymal tumor** |
| • Leiomyoma | |
| • Hemangioma | • Cystic nephroma |
| • Lymphangioma | • Mixed epithelial and stromal tumor |
| • Reninoma | |
| • Fibroma | |
| • Schwannoma | |

the tumor mass. AMLs are also commonly found in women with the rare lung disease lymphangioleiomyomatosis; less commonly they are found in the liver and rarely in other organs.

*Treatment.* Until recently, the treatment for symptomatic AML was either embolization or surgery. The latter is usually reserved for cases with life-threatening bleeding; some experts recommend embolization if the diameter of the AML is greater than 4 cm because of the risk of hemorrhage. Recently, everolimus, a rapamycin derivative that inhibits the mammalian target of rapamycin (mTOR) pathway, has been reported to significantly reduce AML volume in patients with AML and tuberous sclerosis; 42% of patients responded when treated with everolimus versus 0% for placebo.

**Mixed epithelial and mesenchymal tumors** comprise two histologically distinct entities: mixed epithelial and stromal tumors and cystic nephromas. Mixed epithelial and stromal tumors predominantly occur in perimenopausal women, mostly those receiving estrogen therapy. The most common symptoms are flank pain and hematuria, although 25% are asymptomatic. Cystic nephroma is a benign tumor observed predominantly in middle-aged perimenopausal women.

**Renal cell tumors.** Oncocytomas account for approximately 5% of all adult primary renal epithelial neoplasms and 5–15% of surgically resected renal tumors. Most occur sporadically in asymptomatic elderly men. Oncocytomas are typically solitary, well-demarcated, unencapsulated, homogeneous renal cortical tumors. However, bilateral multicentric oncocytomas may be observed in the hereditary syndrome of renal oncocytosis. Oncocytomas are treated by surgical resection.

Papillary adenomas are the most common renal epithelial tumor, often incidentally discovered at postmortem examination. Papillary adenomas are commonly found in elderly patients with acquired renal cystic disease, in patients undergoing long-term hemodialysis and in children with von Hippel–Lindau syndrome. According to the World Health Organizaton (WHO) definition, papillary adenomas are 5 mm or less in diameter, usually subcapsular and solitary. Treatment is by surgical resection.

**Metanephric neoplasms** are a heterogeneous group of benign renal tumors that include metanephric adenoma (epithelial tumor), metanephric stromal tumor (stromal neoplasm) and metanephric adenofibroma (mixed epithelial and stromal neoplasm). These tumors are histogenetically related to Wilm's tumor (see page 127). Metanephric adenomas usually present in the fifth or sixth decade with a 2:1 female preponderance. Metanephric adenomas are asymptomatic in approximately 50% of patients; in those with symptoms, abdominal pain, hematuria and polycythemia are observed.

## Malignant kidney tumors

The most common malignant tumors are renal cell carcinoma and renal pelvic tumors in adults, and Wilm's tumor in children.

**Renal cell carcinomas** are relatively rare and account for only 1–3% of all visceral cancers. They occur most typically in males over 50 years of age. The clinical presentation is variable; tumors may be picked up incidentally or may present with hematuria, loin pain, as a mass or as a paraneoplastic syndrome (hypercalcemia, hypertension or polycythemia). Renal cell cancers often present late and have a relatively poor prognosis. In the absence of metastatic disease, 5-year survival is 70%, but with renal vein involvement or extension into perinephric fat, the 5-year survival is only

20%. Risk factors for renal cell carcinoma include smoking, obesity, acetaminophen (paracetamol) use, gasoline exposure, kidney stones and von Hippel–Lindau disease (approximately 30–50% of all patients).

**Carcinoma of the kidney pelvis** is a transitional cell carcinoma arising from the urothelium. These tumors present early with hematuria or obstruction, and are often associated with similar tumors in the ureters and bladder. Risk factors include a history of analgesic abuse and exposure to aniline dye.

**Wilm's tumors** are the commonest intra-abdominal tumor in children under 10 years of age, with peak incidence between 1 and 4 years. The tumors may contain fibrous tissue, bone and fat. The child may present with an abdominal mass and pain, hematuria, hypertension or intestinal obstruction. Wilm's tumor is aggressive and at the time of diagnosis may have already spread to the lungs.

**Treatment** of renal cell carcinoma is primarily guided by the likelihood of cure, which depends on the stage or degree of tumor dissemination. The therapeutic options are surgery, radiation therapy, chemotherapy, hormonal therapy, immunotherapy, or a combination of these. Only selected patients with metastatic disease respond to immunotherapy, while palliative therapy is the only option in patients with advanced disease, especially if they are elderly. The 2009 American Urologic Association guideline recommends that all therapeutic options should be reviewed with the patient, balancing risk and benefit, as well discussing the impact on kidney function.

*Surgical resection* is recommended for local disease, either by subtotal (partial) or total (radical) nephrectomy. Surgical resection may also be used for palliation in metastatic disease.

*Targeted therapies.* For metastatic disease, the efficacy of chemotherapy and endocrine-based approaches are limited (response rate < 15%), and targeted therapies have now been developed (Table 11.5). Three broad categories of drugs are available:

- mTOR inhibitors
- tyrosine kinase inhibitors
- interleukin (IL)-2.

mTOR inhibitors interfere with the synthesis of proteins that regulate proliferation, growth and survival of tumor cells. Tyrosine kinase inhibitors interfere with both tumor angiogenesis and tumor cell proliferation, resulting in reduced tumor vascularization and cancer cell death, and ultimately tumor shrinkage. IL-2 enhances the proliferation and function of T lymphocytes, which have potent cytotoxic activity against a variety of tumor cells.

TABLE 11.5

**Biological or targeted treatment of renal cell carcinoma***

| Agent | Mechanism of action |
|---|---|
| Everolimus | mTOR inhibitor |
| Bevacizumab | VEGF-A inhibitor |
| Axitinib | Tyrosine kinase inhibitor |
| Sorafenib tosylate | Tyrosine kinase inhibitor |
| Pazopanib hydrochloride | Tyrosine kinase inhibitor |
| Aldesleukin | Interleukin-2 |
| Sunitinib malate | Tyrosine kinase inhibitor |
| Temsirolimus | mTOR inhibitor |

*Drugs approved by the US Food and Drug Administration.
m-TOR, mammalian Target of Rapamycin; VEGF, vascular endothelial growth factor.

**Key points – urinary tract obstruction and tumors**

- Urinary tract obstruction is common and can lead to irreversible kidney failure if not recognized.
- An infected obstructed urinary system is a urologic emergency.
- Renal cell carcinoma often presents late, while transitional cell carcinoma of the kidney pelvis causes obstruction and presents early.
- Targeted therapies are expanding the treatment options for both benign and malignant kidney tumors.

## Key references

Brett AS, Ablin RJ. Prostate-cancer screening – what the U.S. Preventive Services Task Force left out. *N Engl J Med* 2011;365:1949–51.

Chou R, Croswell JM, Dana T et al. Screening for prostate cancer: a review of the evidence for the U.S. Preventive Services Task Force. *Ann Intern Med* 2011;155:762–71.

Cupisti A. Update on nephrolithiasis: beyond symptomatic urinary tract obstruction. *J Nephrol* 2011;24(Suppl 18):S25–9.

Donnell RF. Benign prostate hyperplasia: a review of the year's progress from bench to clinic. *Curr Opin Urol* 2011;21:22–6.

Kirby RS, Gilling PJ. *Fast Facts: Benign Prostatic Hyperplasia*, 7th edn. Oxford: Health Press, 2011.

Kirby RS, Patel MI. *Fast Facts: Prostate Cancer*, 7th edn. Oxford: Health Press, 2012.

Raghavan D, Bailey MJ. *Fast Facts: Bladder Cancer*, 2nd edn. Oxford: Health Press, 2006.

Roehrborn CG. Male lower urinary tract symptoms (LUTS) and benign prostatic hyperplasia (BPH). *Med Clin North Am* 2011;95:87–100.

Three choices for renal replacement therapy are available for patients with end-stage kidney disease (ESKD):

- conservative care and symptom control
- dialysis (either peritoneal or hemodialysis)
- kidney transplant (from a living or cadaveric donor).

In general, all patients should be offered all suitable choices, and be fully counseled as to the advantages and disadvantages of each. In reality, however, not all options are available in all centers, and patient-related factors can be limiting.

### Conservative care

Dialysis may not improve quality of life in patients with extensive comorbidities. Indeed, there is some evidence that very elderly patients, with only limited comorbid illnesses, may not even have the length of their lives prolonged by dialysis. In these circumstances, many patients opt for symptom control without dialysis, using erythropoietin, vitamin D analogs, dietary control, antipruritics and antiemetics as necessary. Such patients often have significantly better quality of life, fewer hospital admissions (e.g. from dialysis-related complications), and are more likely to die finally at home rather than in hospital than patients receiving dialysis.

Conservative care does not represent an absence of renal support, but rather the active medical (non-technological) management of the complications of kidney failure. It is clearly important that patients participate fully in these discussions wherever possible. A multidisciplinary team approach is crucial and should involve nurses, doctors, counselors and family members.

### Dialysis

The term dialysis refers to the physical process of the diffusion of a molecule down its concentration gradient, from an area of high concentration to an area of lower concentration, through a semipermeable membrane.

Hemodialysis involves pumping blood from the body through an artificial kidney in which the blood is surrounded by a solution of electrolytes, called the dialysate, the concentration of which can be varied precisely. Solutes present in the blood at high concentration (e.g. urea, potassium, creatinine) diffuse into the dialysate and are removed (Figure 12.1).

Changing the concentration of solutes in the dialysate can alter the electrolyte composition of the blood. Raising the dialysate calcium above the serum concentration, for example, can increase serum calcium in patients with hypocalcemia.

A separate biophysical process, ultrafiltration, is used to regulate the distribution of water between the blood and dialysate. The volume of water to be removed from the patient's blood can be controlled by altering the pressures on either side of the membrane separating the blood from the dialysate.

The dialysis machine itself is simply the housing for the pumps controlling blood and dialysate flow, various safety devices (pressure sensors, air detectors), a system for maintaining blood anticoagulation in the extracorporeal circuit (usually a heparin infusion), and a screen for graphically displaying the various parameters monitored. Different modalities of dialysis differ in the precise balance of ultrafiltration and dialysis, the speed of blood flow and the nature of the dialysate.

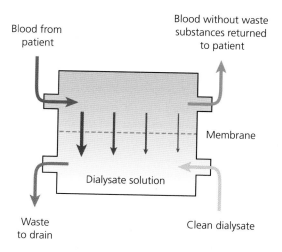

**Figure 12.1** The principle of hemodialysis.

TABLE 12.1

**Complications of hemodialysis**

| Access related | Complications during hemodialysis |
|---|---|
| • Local infection | • Hypotension |
| • Sepsis and bacteremia | • Cardiac arrhythmias |
| • Endocarditis and osteomyelitis | • Nausea and vomiting |
| • Fistula stenosis or thrombosis | • Headache |
| | • Cramps |
| • Superior vena cava, subclavian or internal jugular vein stenosis | • Fever |
| | • Allergic reactions (e.g. to dialysers, tubing) |
| • Fistula aneurysm formation | • Air embolism |
| | • Heparin-induced thrombocytopenia |
| | • Seizures |
| | • Hemolysis |

Patients need excellent vascular access, and access problems are a major cause of morbidity (Table 12.1). Access is obtained through either a fistula created between a peripheral artery and vein (usually radial or brachial), or a permanent plastic catheter inserted into an internal jugular or subclavian vein (Figure 12.2).

Hemodialysis can be carried out in a main hospital center, a satellite unit (often staffed only by nurses) or in the patient's home. Home hemodialysis offers patients the most autonomy, but requires a suitable house with a water supply, space (for the machine and supplies), a reasonably technically competent patient and usually a trained helper who will be present during each dialysis session. Patients dialysing at home often have the best quality of life. Dialysis is usually performed three times each week for about 4 hours. Some patients opt for daily hemodialysis (usually 6 days/week), which provides the best control of fluid balance and biochemistry, but is intensive. Patients can dialyse overnight while they sleep either at home or in dialysis centers. It is difficult to determine the optimum amount of dialysis a patient requires, and various methods are in use.

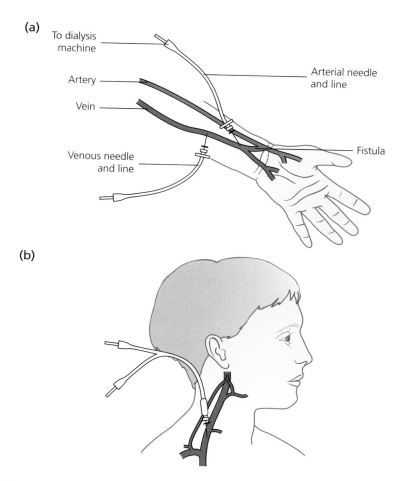

**Figure 12.2** (a) Forearm arteriovenous fistula for hemodialysis; (b) internal jugular catheter for hemodialysis.

**Peritoneal dialysis** uses the peritoneal cavity as a reservoir into which a dialysate can be infused, and the blood flowing through peritoneal capillaries as the blood source. Dialysis and ultrafiltration occur across these capillaries. Ultrafiltration is controlled by altering the osmolality of the dialysate solution and thus drawing water out of the patient's blood. This can be achieved with glucose or other large-molecular-weight solutes in the dialysate. The glucose load can cause problems of its own, such as poor diabetic control and weight gain.

Dialysate is infused through a catheter, which is inserted into the patient's peritoneum under local or general anesthetic and remains in place permanently. The waste solutes are removed by exchanging the peritoneal fluid for a fresh solution (Figure 12.3). As long as patients have reasonable manual dexterity, they can be trained to perform continuous ambulatory peritoneal dialysis, typically four exchanges spaced throughout the day with each one taking about 20 minutes, or to use a machine (automated peritoneal dialysis) to do a number of exchanges overnight while they sleep, and then perform only one or two daytime exchanges.

Peritoneal dialysis is carried out by the patient at home, at work or while on holiday. It therefore allows the patient a high degree of independence and control over their own illness. However, patients must not be allowed to become isolated, and still need considerable support.

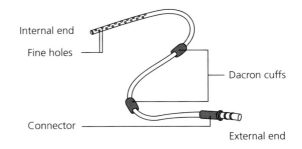

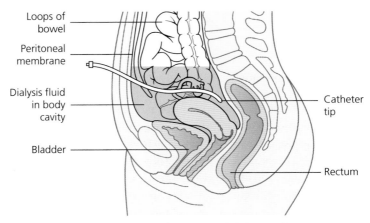

**Figure 12.3** Design and position of a peritoneal dialysis catheter.

Intra-abdominal adhesions and abdominal wall stoma are absolute contraindications for peritoneal dialysis, and obesity, intestinal disease, respiratory disease and hernias are relative contraindications. The complications of peritoneal dialysis are listed in Table 12.2.

**When to start dialysis.** The question of when to start dialysis remains controversial. In general, patients should begin dialysis when estimated glomerular filtration rate (GFR) is in the range of 8–10 mL/minute/1.73m². There is no good evidence that starting dialysis earlier is of any benefit to patients. If dialysis is delayed for too long, however, patients can become very malnourished. Nevertheless, there are excellent data suggesting that earlier referral for nephrological care before renal replacement therapy is required can significantly delay the need for dialysis, and reduce early morbidity and mortality.

**Dialysis and pregnancy.** Most women with ESKD on dialysis are infertile, and pregnancy is extremely uncommon. Fertility often returns rapidly after a successful kidney transplant (see below). If women on dialysis do become pregnant, the outcome is usually poor with a very high risk of miscarriage, severe hypertension, small babies and prematurity. Only 47% of women have a successful obstetric outcome.

## Transplantation

A kidney transplant provides the best long-term outcome for patients with ESKD. A transplant can come from a cadaveric donor, from a living

TABLE 12.2

**Complications of peritoneal dialysis**

- Peritonitis
- Catheter infection
- Catheter blockage, kinking, leaks or slow drainage
- Constipation
- Fluid retention
- Hyperglycemia
- Weight gain
- Hernias (incisional, inguinal, umbilical)
- Back pain
- Malnutrition
- Encapsulating peritoneal sclerosis (rare)

relative or from an unrelated living donor (often called emotionally related). The sale of organs for transplantation is prohibited in almost all countries, but nevertheless continues, mostly because of the severe shortage of organs. All patients with ESKD should be considered for a transplant. Age itself is not a major determinant of outcome, though the presence of comorbid disease adversely affects survival (Table 12.3).

Patients should be aware of the risks and benefits of transplantation (Table 12.4), and require screening for occult cardiovascular disease before

TABLE 12.3

**Contraindications for transplantation**

- Cancer
- Active infection
- Uncontrolled ischemic heart disease
- Aquired immunodeficiency disease with opportunistic infections

- Active viral hepatitis
- Extensive peripheral vascular disease
- Mental incapacity

TABLE 12.4

**Risks and benefits of kidney transplantation**

| Risks | Benefits |
|---|---|
| • Immediate operative complications (local infection, pain, pneumonia, deep-vein thrombosis) | • Cessation of dialysis |
| • Immediate graft failure | • Improved quality of life |
| • Arterial or venous thrombosis in the transplant | • Reversal of anemia |
| • Infections (viral, bacterial, fungal) | • Reversal of kidney bone disease |
| • Cancer (skin, lymphoma) | • Normalization of diet |
| • Side effects of immunosuppressive drugs (common) | • Relaxation of fluid restriction |
| • Death at time of surgery (rare) | |

surgery. Over 90% of transplants should be working 1 year after surgery. A cadaveric transplant should have a mean survival of 15 years and a living transplant about 18–20 years.

Patients do not generally have their native kidneys removed, and the transplanted kidney is placed extraperitoneally in the iliac fossa. Patients can usually expect to stay in hospital for 1–3 weeks, and require frequent follow-up after discharge (two or three times each week initially).

Patients will be treated with a cocktail of immunosuppressant drugs, which may include ciclosporin, azathioprine, mycophenolate mofetil, tacrolimus, sirolimus or prednisolone. These drugs must be taken for life and require careful monitoring (Table 12.5). Patients will also have received potent immunosuppression at the time of surgery, including monoclonal antibodies against the interleukin-2 (IL-2) receptor or T lymphocytes, or antithymocyte globulin.

**Common complications.** Routine postoperative problems, such as deep-vein thrombosis, pulmonary embolism and pneumonia, can occur. Specific problems include opportunistic infections (viral, fungal, bacterial), malignancies (especially skin cancers), drug toxicity, recurrence of the original disease in the transplant, cardiovascular disease, hypertension, dyslipidemia and graft failure (Table 12.6). Patients should be followed up for life and undergo annual screening for cancers, drug toxicity and cardiovascular disease in addition to routine clinic visits. Most patients with a transplant will die from cardiovascular disease, which should, therefore, be aggressively managed.

Fertility is usually restored in women after a kidney transplant, but transplant recipients have a high risk of hypertension during pregnancy, and an increased risk of miscarriage in the first trimester and premature delivery. Some immunosuppressants (e.g. mycophenolate mofetil) also pose a risk to the fetus.

TABLE 12.5

## Side effects of immunosuppressant drugs

### All drugs

- Increased risk of infections
- Increased risk of malignancy (especially skin cancer and lymphoma)

### Prednisolone

- Diabetes
- Osteoporosis
- Weight gain
- Hypertension
- Poor wound healing

### Ciclosporin

- Hyperkalemia
- Tremor
- Neuropathy
- Hirsutism
- Nephrotoxicity
- Hypertension
- Dyslipidemia
- Gingival hypertrophy

### Mycophenolate mofetil

- Diarrhea
- Constipation
- Nausea
- Leukopenia, anemia, thrombocytopenia

### Azathioprine

- Hypersensitivity reactions
- Bone marrow suppression
- Hepatotoxicity
- Hair loss
- Colitis and pancreatitis

### Tacrolimus

- Gastrointestinal disturbance
- Nephrotoxicity
- Hypertension
- Tremor
- Hirsutism
- Dyslipidemia
- Diabetes

### Sirolimus

- Hyperlipidemia
- Thrombocytopenia
- Leukopenia
- Mouth ulcers
- Poor wound healing

TABLE 12.6

**Complications of kidney transplantation**

| Complication | Prevention | Management |
|---|---|---|
| **Early (days)** | | |
| Immediate surgical complications | Heparin, wound care, physiotherapy | As normal |
| Urinary infection | | Early detection and treatment |
| **1–4 weeks** | | |
| Viral infections (especially herpes simplex virus) | Aciclovir prophylaxis | Aciclovir |
| Graft rejection | Immunosuppression drug monitoring | Corticosteroids, adjust immunosuppression |
| Acute tubular necrosis | Blood pressure control, fluid balance | Treat cause |
| Ciclosporin nephrotoxicity | Immunosuppression drug monitoring | Immunosuppression drug monitoring |
| Urinary obstruction | Ureteric stent insertion | Early detection, cystoscopy, stent |
| **Later** | | |
| Opportunistic infections | Avoid over-immunosuppression | Treat infection aggressively |
| Rejection | Immunosuppression drug monitoring | Corticosteroids, adjust immunosuppression |
| Ciclosporin nephrotoxicity | Immunosuppression drug monitoring | Immunosuppression drug monitoring |
| Bone marrow suppression | Avoid overimmuno-suppression, monitor with complete blood count | Reduce drug dose, may need bone marrow examination |
| Cytomegalovirus infection | Ganciclovir prophylaxis | Ganciclovir |
| Lymphoma | Avoid overimmuno-suppression | Reduce drug doses; may need chemotherapy |

## Key points – renal replacement therapy and transplantation

- Not all patients with end-stage kidney disease (ESKD) need or want dialysis, and some may be managed conservatively.
- Most patients will require several modalities of renal replacement therapy in their lifetime.
- Hemodialysis requires excellent vascular access; problems with access cause significant morbidity.
- Peritoneal dialysis is an excellent modality for many patients, especially early in ESKD.
- Transplantation offers the best long-term outcomes, but at the expense of long-term side effects from immunosuppression, including cancers and cardiovascular disease.
- Most women on dialysis are infertile. Fertility is restored after transplantation, but pregnant transplant recipients have an increased risk of hypertension, miscarriage in the first trimester and premature delivery.

### Key references

Heemann U, Abramowicz D, Spasovski G, Vanholder R; European Renal Best Practice Work Group on Kidney Transplantation. Endorsement of the Kidney Disease Improving Global Outcomes (KDIGO) guidelines on kidney transplantation: a European Renal Best Practice (ERBP) position statement. *Nephrol Dial Transplant* 2011;26:2099–106.

Locatelli F, Cavalli A, Viganò SM, Pontoriero G. Lessons from recent trials on hemodialysis. *Contrib Nephrol* 2011;171:30–8.

Lunsford KE, Barbas AS, Brennan TV. Recent advances in immunosuppressive therapy for prevention of renal allograft rejection. *Curr Opin Organ Transplant* 2011;16:390–7.

Metalidis C, Kuypers DR. Emerging immunosuppressive drugs in kidney transplantation. *Curr Clin Pharmacol* 2011;6:130–6.

Sprangers B, Kuypers DR, Vanrenterghem Y. Immunosuppression: does one regimen fit all? *Transplantation* 2011;92:251–61.

# Useful resources

**UK**
British Renal Society
www.britishrenal.org

British Transplantation Society
www.bts.org.uk

The Kidney Alliance
www.kidneyalliance.org

Kidney Patient Guide
www.kidneypatientguide.org.uk

National Kidney Federation
www.kidney.org.uk

The Renal Association
www.renal.org

UK Renal Registry
www.renalreg.com

**USA**
American Association of Kidney
Patients
www.aakp.org

American Society of Nephrology
www.asn-online.org

The Kidney Trust
http://kidneytrust.org

National Kidney Foundation
www.kidney.org

Nephron Information Center
http://nephron.com

**International**
Australian and New Zealand
Society of Nephrology
www.nephrology.edu.au

Canadian Society of Nephrology
www.csnscn.ca/en

Kidney Foundation of Canada
www.kidney.ca

Kidney Health Australia
www.kidney.org.au

International Federation of
Kidney Foundations
www.ifkf.org

International Society of
Nephrology
www.theisn.org

Renal Society of Australasia
www.renalsociety.org

Other useful websites
www.patientpictures.com/urology
www.renalinfo.com

# Index